# THE ULTIMATE GUIDE TO
# Tantric SEX

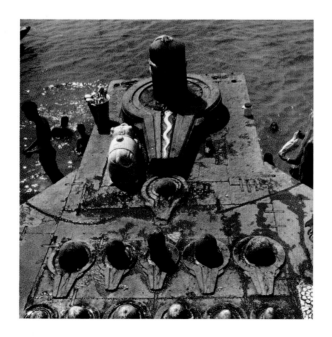

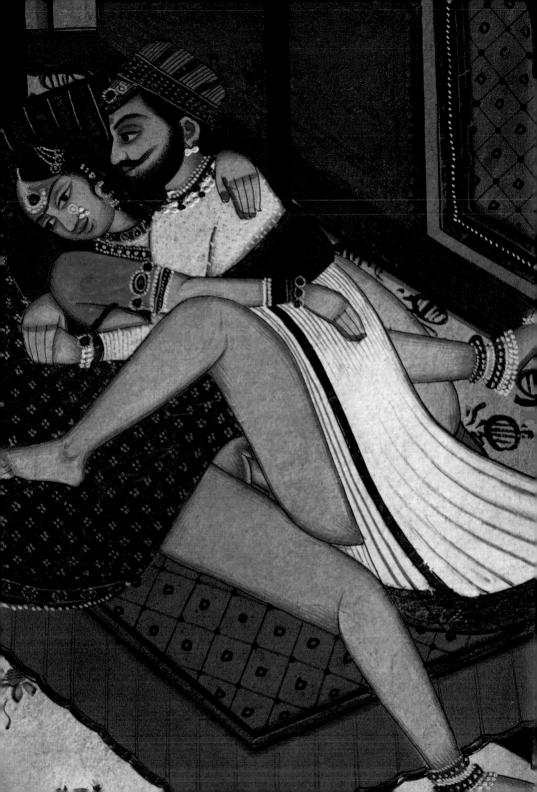

# THE ULTIMATE GUIDE TO
# Tantric SEX

## Guillermo Ferrara

### 19 Lessons to Achieving Ecstasy

Translated by William Haynes

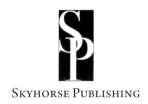

SKYHORSE PUBLISHING

DISCLAIMER: This book offers suggestions only, and in no way should it be used as a substitute for consultation with professional therapists. The information provided in this work offers you the knowledge so you can choose, at your own risk, to act on that knowledge.

Original Title: Lecciones de Sexo Tántrico

© 2004, Guillermo Ferrara

© 2004, 2005, Editorial Océano, S.L.

(Barcelona, Spain)

Photos: Becky Lawton, M & G Studios, Stock Photos, AGE Fotostock, Amber Ocean Stock

Drawings: Xavier Bou

Models: Guillermo Ferrara, Eliana Alonso, Selena Leo, Leonardo Valley, Sandra Sentíes, Enrique Ojeda, Sonia Soler, Eduard Mundi, Ricard Pons, Belinda Baldiw

Props courtesy of The Company of China, Aquamarine Services

Skyhorse Publishing books may be purchased in bulk at special discounts for sales promotion, corporate gifts, fund-raising, or educational purposes. Special editions can also be created to specifications. For details, contact the Special Sales Department, Skyhorse Publishing, 307 West 36th Street, 11th Floor, New York, NY 10018 or info@skyhorsepublishing.com.

Skyhorse® and Skyhorse Publishing® are registered trademarks of Skyhorse Publishing, Inc.®, a Delaware corporation.

Visit our website at www.skyhorsepublishing.com.

10 9 8 7 6 5 4 3

Library of Congress Cataloging-in-Publication Data is available on file.

Cover design by Qualcom

Cover photo credit courtesy of Océano Ambar

ISBN: 978-1-63220-327-4

Ebook ISBN: 978-1-63220-860-6

Printed in China

"There is a Brotherhood of Tantrics waiting to be brought to life. This brotherhood will awaken as the end of the Kali Age approaches. Recognizing the potent female principle of life, the brotherhood of Tantra will transform this corrupted world. Then, at the ecstatic moment when one age transforms into the next, those faithful followers of the selfless path will reach their goal."

KAULA TANTRA

### Dedication

*To Sandra. Your beautiful presence in this space and time built a home inside of me. You are a magical woman, a gift of life.*

# Contents

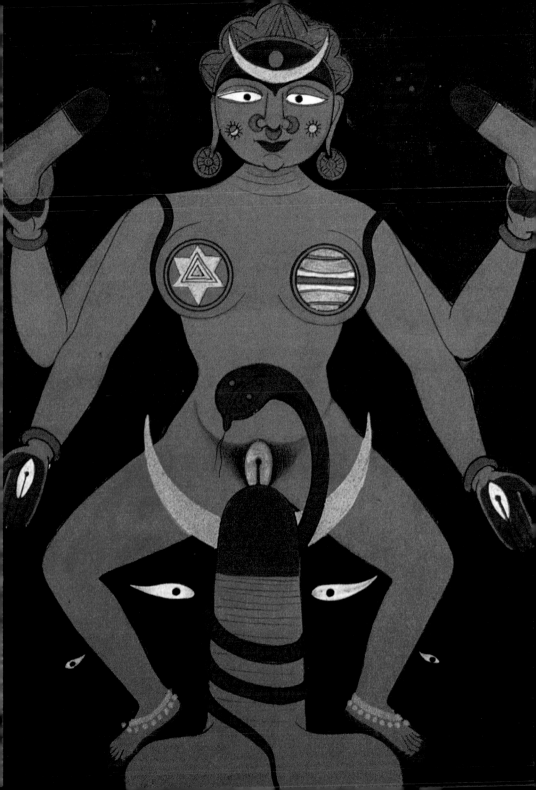

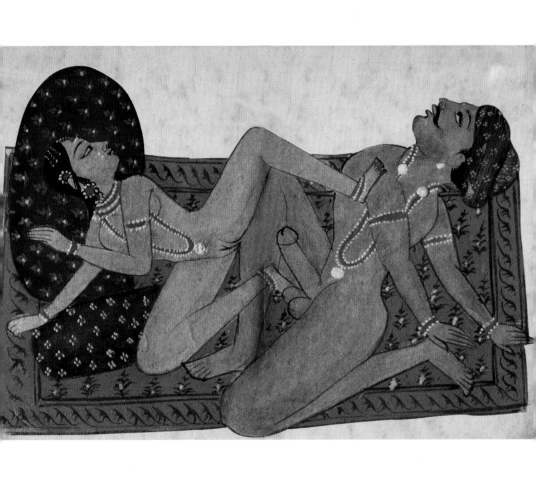

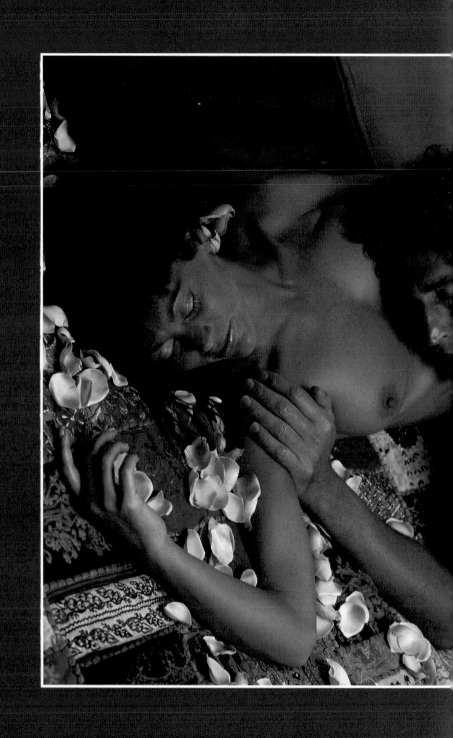

# What is Tantra?

*"Sex is man's most vital energy
and should not be an end to itself.
Sex should guide man to his soul.
The objective: from lust until light."*

OSHO

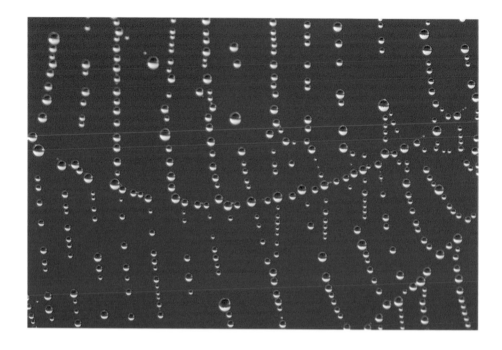

**Tantra integrates the brightest values of life: power and conscious energy, the basic pillars in which they flow.**

Tantra is an existential compendium for discovering the vital road leading to spiritual evolution through beauty, art, love, meditation, joy, and meditative sex. It dates back to the dark ages, in ancient India, where Shiva (the god) revealed the secrets of life to his consort Shakti (the goddess), also called Parvati.

It is also a method for growth that allows an evolving practice in all aspects of one's individuality: wealth, sexuality, nutrition, art, love, creativity, perception through internal intuition and mysticism, and spiritual power.

For the tantric, we are not fragmented nor divided; there are many people who feel it, so it is also an integrative, comprehensive, and free way to heal deteriorating mental conditions, taboos, and old emotional wounds.

In fact, the word "Tantra" is composed of "tan" ("tissues") and "tra" ("release"); etymologically it comes from "tanoti" ("expansion") and "trayoti" ("release"). It is a vital tissue that connects all facets of a human to a divine, spiritual liberation.

Tantra shows life as an inexhaustible tissue where situations, people, events, and experiences are intertwined so that, with each other, we can come together towards a full development, both personal and collective.

The "Tantras" are also the ancient, sacred books that mention the secrets and techniques to achieve spiritual enlightenment. Tantra seeks the same goal, but not as obsessively. During this personal journey, it is enjoyed without mortification but with rejoicing, meditation, abundant laughter and love, and intelligence. In fact, consciousness and energy go hand in hand as the perfect formula for progress. To expand this awareness of life, there is an emphasis on raising one's energy.

Although there are several sacred texts, the ancient tantric passed down an oral tradition that is difficult to access; learning was primarily through direct experience.

without performing sex; the second is fully immersed in sexual practices, rituals, and the encouragement of the **kundalini** energy.

This book is inspired by the Hindu Tantra and its intention is nothing more than to share life and the secrets of sexual experience so men and women today can manage their sexual energy and improve their spiritual evolution.

These methods are not a religion, nor do they imply power structures, but are a clear invitation to direct learning, without the need for intermediaries. Although Tantra is practiced as a couple (whether casual lovers or committed couples), it also moves to increase the spiritual fire, energy of attraction, seduction, and sensuality as well as to practice yoga, massages, rituals, symbols, mantras, and sex.

**Shiva**
or "The Supreme Danzarin," one of the three aspects (along with Brahma and Vishnu) of the divine trinity of Hinduism. Alongside is the goddess Kali.

## Two roads

In Tantra, there are two basic methods: Buddhist Tantra, or **right hand**, and Hindu Tantra, or **left hand**. The first emphasizes **meditation** and contemplation

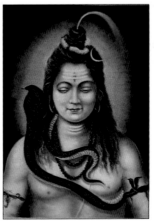

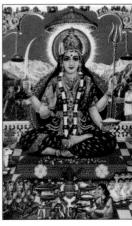

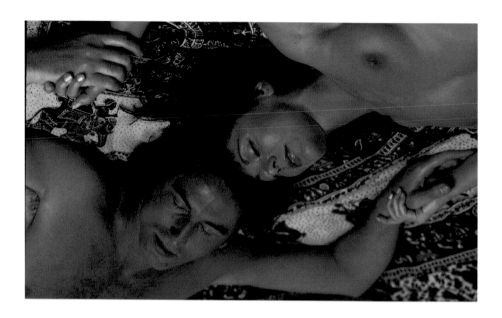

**In the West, Tantra is popular because it includes sexual activity among those who practice it.**

Tantra has become popular in the West because its methods involve personal practices for sexual activity. The drawback is that many of its students begin to think about eating dessert before the main course; the maithuna, or sexual rite, is the last piece after the practices in energy, or sadhana.

Regardless, the vision of Tantra moves beyond mere sex or pleasure (that can be obtained in unlimited quantities). Instead, it points towards an understanding that the universe is a constant, creative whole balanced by two fundamental energies: Shiva and Shakti, the male and female poles.

These poles, these principles, are both the macrocosm and microcosm: a human being is a small-scale mirror of the whole of humanity. It is easy to see that this vision opens a huge and bright set of vital possibilities.

## Shiva and Shakti

Understand that in the beginning, we were whole; the idea of "one" was not expressed before the Big Bang. From this creation arises a duality of the two opposite and complementary poles: the female, Shakti, and the male, Shiva. Shakti and Shiva coexist, forming a permanent equilibrium in the universe.

Shiva is the light, the cosmic Danzarin, the main solar, and male consciousness. Shakti is the goddess, consort of Shiva, his love, Parvati; she is also the dark night, the energy, the Great Mother, the power of creation, fertilization, female, woman, sister, priestess, lover.

In the beginning, Shiva and Shakti were **androgynous**, united by the same energy. Through sex, these two forces were released to the universe to create life and maintain balance between the two poles. The tantric sex act aims to feel the fusion of the two gods within us; when a woman and a man gaze deep into each other's being, it is not just an invitation to pleasure and to love, but a transcendent unity of these poles that govern life.

The tantric sex ritual, **maithuna**, joins Shiva and Shakti in any man or woman who feel the divine identity through the **lingam** (the male sexual organ) and the **yoni** (the vagina, the gate of life). This union of Tantra is much more than a physical event; it also opens the doors for creation and the raw material that founded life: pleasure, consciousness, energy, motion, and beauty.

Tantric practice seeks nothing less than to embody the divinity of Shiva and Shakti in our consciousness, to feel the sacred character through our sexual encounters, laughter, teaching, dancing, and the revelation of the secrets of life. Every being has its Shiva and Shakti within; you can find the essence of each within both male and female bodies beyond the limits of personality.

The union of the bodies through sex is the ability to perceive the primary unit of the androgynous, a mindless moment, without identification, without limitation, a meeting of the same light, consciousness, the supreme delight, the reunion with the origin of life itself.

According to the theory of Panspermia, Earth was "fertilized" (like an egg) by a comet. This was the birth of life as we know it.

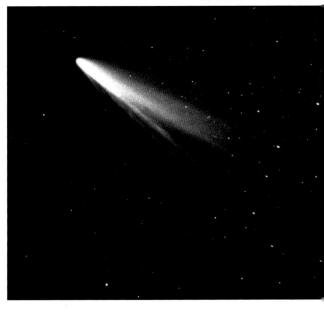

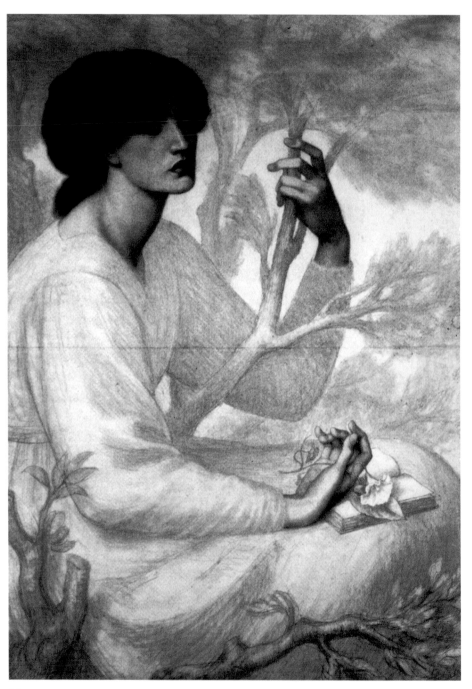

# Ardhanarisvara: the androgynous

*"The symbol of sex also expresses the reality of love. True love represents a relationship, but the word 'love' (like the word 'sex') is used thoughtlessly and without considering its true meaning. Love and sex are fundamentally the same thing, because both express the meaning of the Law of Attraction. Sex is sex and love is love because both words are equally represented in a relationship: interaction, union between god and his universe, man and god, man and his own soul, and between man and woman. This highlights the basis of the relationship. But the result of that relationship is the creation and manifestation of the way through which divinity can express itself and grow."*

Sex, by ALICE BAILEY AND DJWHAL KHUL

Before the creation of dual energy (Shiva and Shakti, ying and yang, male and female), before the Big Bang, there was an original unity. The Supreme Divinity's overflow of ecstasy gave rise to the movement of life within the dual manifestation.

The androgynous Tantra comes from the beginning of humanity. Then, through sex (from the Latin "sectus" meaning "cut" or "split"), humanity was divided into woman and man willing to play the Game of Life, or **Lilah**, to meet again in a countless number of personalities and forms.

This includes a cosmic game that we must learn to play. Through the energy of sex and love, we become

One again. **Ardhanarisvara** is half man and half woman. Every being is androgynous with an inclination towards being more masculine or feminine. Women have small amounts of testosterone and men have small amounts of estrogen. Today, we can see this androgyny in urban fashion trends as well as in people.

It is really erotic to see people balance these two polarities. This does not mean effeminate men or masculine women, but women who feel the attraction of other women with extreme sensuality and femininity, just as men generate an energy of brotherhood and friendship.

The man holds a woman's internal kundalini shakti personified in his sexual, spiritual energy, and

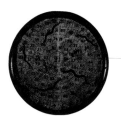

Original Hindu tablet for the game of Lilah ("Snakes and Ladders").

**When a woman has an orgasm, the man should completely identify with her.**

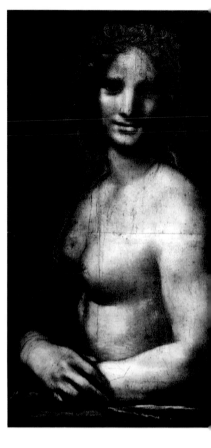

**In certain moments, Shiva becomes more passive, as open as a flower.**

when a woman of flesh and blood arrives with her vibrations, his inner woman is excited. The power of Shakti is the energy of life that, once ignited, expands consciousness, opens doors, and breaks chains in order to slip into the skin of one who feels pure eroticism, an ancestral and sexual energy.

Man has to find the woman inside himself in order to be at peace with himself. It may be done alone and then followed by the reflection offered through his mistress.

Tantra neither promotes nor condemns sex shared with multiple people (it is a personal decision), but considers this attraction as natural and inevitable. If you feel (albeit unknown) that someone stimulates your androgynous inside, it is a basic invitation to this experience.

Sex is a natural phenomenon (nude, metaphysical, and transcendental) that far exceeds the mental virus that has infected humanity. It's a big wave that cannot be stopped. In these times, the androgynous tide comes in hard to demystify sexual misconceptions. A woman's inner love intensifies her man, thus intensifying their shared enthusiasm. When a woman has an orgasm, the man must be fully identified with her, being united and communing with the supreme delight. When Shakti releases their orgasmic power, Shiva absorbs it as a gift from the gods. A multiorgasmic woman maintains a balance of their inner androgynous; it is a miracle of contemporary nature.

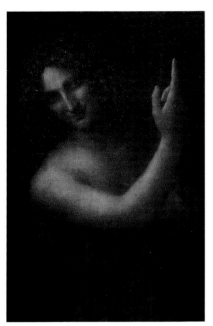
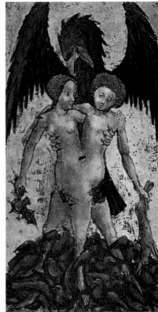

The artistic representation of androgyny clarifies the common origin of the man and the woman.

When this vibrant current comes into action, all of the woman's systems are revitalized, especially the seven chakras that make up the human psyche, which can achieve dimensions well beyond the ordinary sense. This ecstatic union is a return on the direct road to the divine. The ego that keeps a person dissolved and in conflict disappears until it becomes naked and spiritual, under a roof made of the universe: stars, worlds, and wisdom.

The woman awakens in the man an inner woman, a reflection of his wife, in the same way a man is reflected in every woman who feels attracted to her inner man, which occurs naturally and is not condemned in any kind of relationship.

It occurs naturally, specifically during a sexual act. Both man and woman have active and passive roles, just like how, at certain times, Shiva will become passive and as open as a flower while Shakti will become active like a steed of orgasmic energy.

**Sex is a natural phenomenon (nude, metaphysical, and transcendental) that far exceeds the mental virus that has infected humanity.**

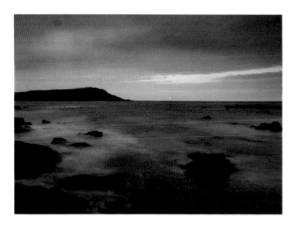

**During its initial appearance, the practice of Tantra will have positive, real results when there is previous work freeing the ego and creating a greater flow of light on the cells and the soul.**

# The magic path of sexual energy

*"Where there is ecstasy, there is creation;*
*where there is no ecstasy, there is no creation;*
*In the infinite, there is ecstasy.*
*There is no ecstasy in the finite."*
CHANDOGYA UPANISHAD

Tantra channels a known sexual energy. As is already known, the first stage of a sexual encounter is pleasure. What is not known is that sexual energy can create a **magical act**. Do not be alarmed; as Coelho says, "Magic is the bloodstream of the universe."

To simply imagine, we don't have to do anything to use a mental, magical energy. Sometimes we imagine situations or negative events, but these are only products of our minds. The idea is to imagine something on the mental plane and then perform it in the real world, just like creative people do. Tantra uses this energy, the potential enormous amounts of energy, or intent, during sex, to make a leap to focus on a single point.

In other words, sex generates an awareness of this power that can be focused towards an intent. As Shiva and Shakti, as with every man and woman, we are co-creators with the universal creator; sex is the pure energy of creation. This immense strength and power channels through the law that says "Energy follows thought."

Before their sexual rituals, couples decide on their intentions in order to promote that particular magical and living encounter. Then, through certain mantras, sexual positions, and certain "body bolts," they can accumulate energy, the creative power of sexual will towards a particular purpose.

In this specific part of this book, you will see how you can use the magical aspect of this energy to rise above the level of animal instinct and increase the flow of light, magic, and surprise in your life.

# Khajuraho: the temples of love

This enigmatic, sensual, and artistic place in India is a relic of the golden age of the East. For centuries, Khujuraho has exhibited the majesty and beauty of sex.

To the ancients, sex was a vehicle, a means to express the supreme. And they saw in bodies a treasure, a place to manifest physical and spiritual fulfillment. This town in India has become famous for its temples containing stone etchings of countless sexual positions and styles.

These monuments from thousands of years ago celebrate an erotic art, a culture that viewed the natural in all of its forms. They teach us the art of love. Somehow, through different sexual positions, energy is able to flow more intensely through the chakras and illuminate the seventh chakra at the top of the head.

These sculptures reflect that eternity is connected to the sexual act (and all present acts); only sex can increase the perceptual capacity.

Ancient artists created authentic works of stone art.

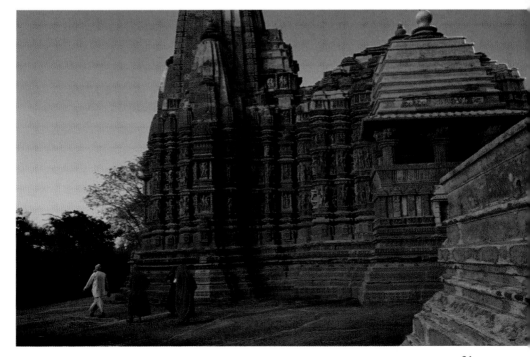

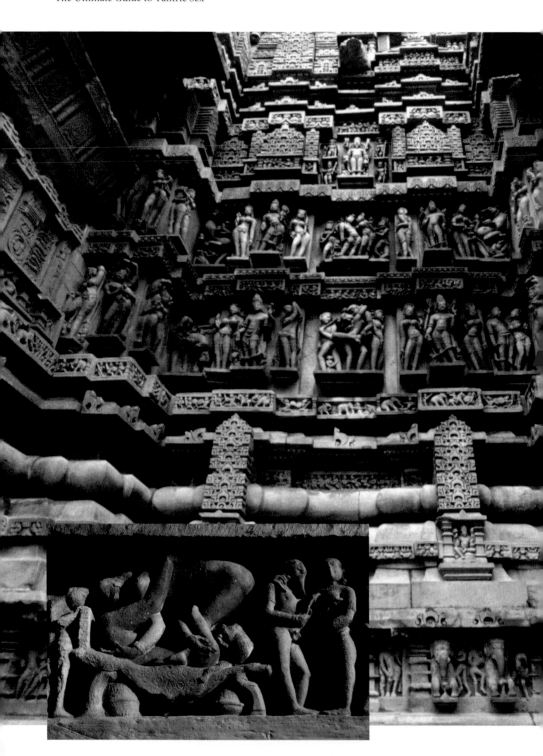

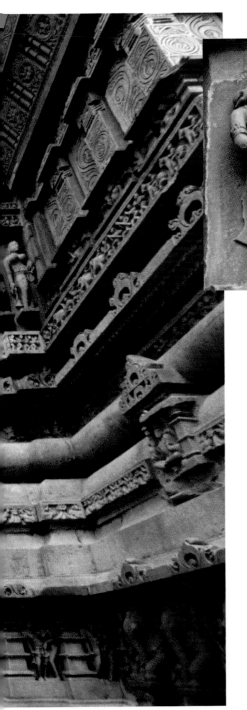

Unlike other spiritual roads, Tantra reflects the abundance and wealth in all forms. God is rich and life is abundant and we get to immerse ourselves in that consciousness. The time Khajuraho was constructed, it reflected the golden light and splendor of Eastern wisdom.

In Tantra, when one overflows this energy, it is reflected as art and seeks to reflect the worship of the principles of life. In Tantra, life is sex. The varieties of sculptures show couples connecting with two or more partners. A moralistic look may see this as perverse, but for Tantra, it is an observation of the freedom beyond the ordinary personality,

**It seeks to worship the beginning of life. For Tantra, life is sex.**

23

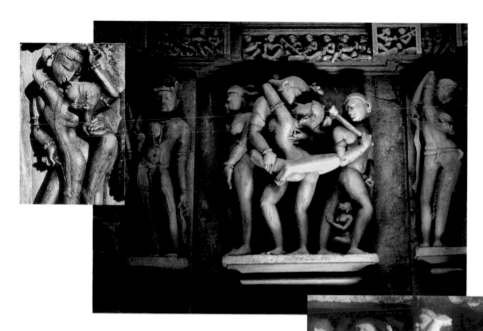

**In 1986, this assembly of temples was called "Heritage of Humanity."** ego, jealousy, and anything that soils desire and love. The chains and shackles of censorship are in the mind, forever oxidized along with sexual repression. When these are broken, then one may really see the beautiful images of Khajuraho.

The sexual sculptures are found on the outside of the temple while there are no pictures inside so that one may enter with an open heart and mind.

Many sculptures refer to not only sexual positions, but the art of the kiss, hug, and even gaze. If you look at the images without thinking, you see innocence, pleasure, and ease. In the time of Vatsyayana, the author of *Kama Sutra*, there was an emphasis on the art of love that helped build a perfect state of inner peace and fulfillment. There are currently many new editions of the *Kama Sutra* in many different styles. In some schools of thought, there is a subject called "love" or "meditative sex."

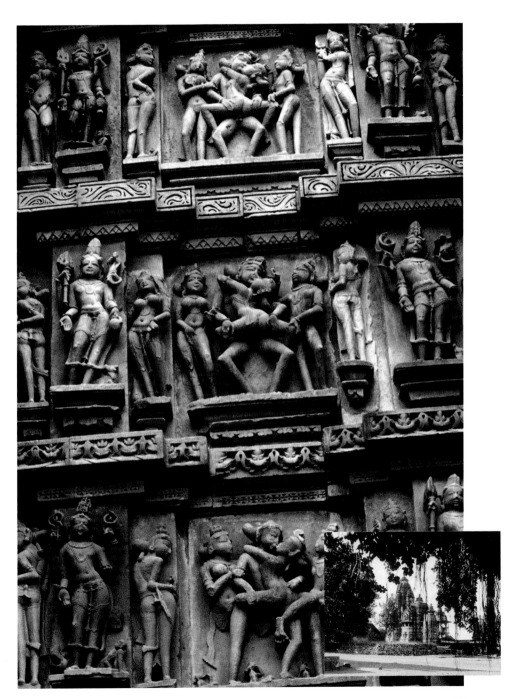

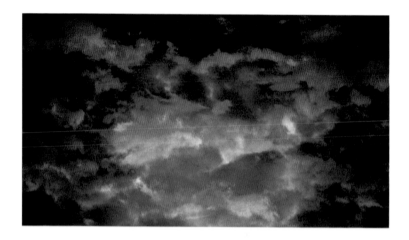

# Basics of tantric sex

There can be sex without love; this is something completely natural; it is the inevitable end of attraction. While there are religions that blindly attempt to segregate these two poles, there is a natural and invisible call that cannot be stopped.

Therefore, if there is attraction and the spark is ignited, this can cause a fire. Often, there is a spark of attraction before the fire of love. This isn't a bad thing, but a natural part of life. You can definitely have sex without love because love always comes as a surprise!

What is the difference between traditional sex and tantric sex? Essentially, it's the attitude and the use of energy. Consciousness is placed on a higher plane. It is like the difference between what an ant sees and what an eagle sees. The ant only sees a portion. Instinctive sex aims to drown tensions, anxiety, and repression. The eagle, on the other hand, represents the tantric couple. Its vision and consciousness is expanded; it doesn't just see the mountains, but the valleys, rivers, and trees; it can see the entire landscape.

There is a huge difference between an ordinary relationship and a tantric one. Tantra awakens the inner eye through special practice. In the first phase we experience only instinctive sex, but later can fly to heavens of ecstasy through meditative sexual practice.

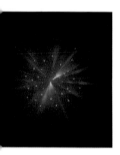

**Many times, a spark of attraction comes first, then the fire of love.**

## The psychology of tantric love

Love is an elevated energy. When we tell others the good news of meeting someone special, we say, "I felt a rush," and when that energy depletes, we say that we are at a "low." These changes of power show that we are emotional and sensitive beings.

Love is a state of consciousness, an awakened set of potentials and qualities. Interestingly, during the tantric exercise of yoga, this energy rises, thus raising the state of love. When this energy rises, consciousness expands, and upon expanding it also creates what we call love. This love is not a state that is necessarily addressed at someone in particular, but is diffused in all directions. The sun provides energy to the entire world. The flowers give away their scent freely without distinction and allow their bees to benefit from their nectar.

Likewise, tantric love awakens anyone who wants to try it, anyone who wants an impact on their heart, a shift in consciousness, or just a pleasureful meeting.

Learning from nature, we can see that everything has beautiful, loving energy. The ultimate teaching of Tantra is to let this love fill our entire being, the surrender to All, Mahamudra, the great symbol of love. As we progress in our spiritual journey, this state increases; it arises from meditation, explores our very essence, and wants to be discovered. The entire mystery of the inner path consists of waiting for the moment of

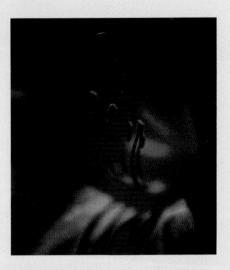

the Big Bang of love, the illumination of the soul. When we look in the existential mirror and see the face of the divine, that face is known as universal love. We proceed through the Light— it is our beginning and we have come to this Earth to play among the shadows. Thus, when we open the inner door of our hearts, we are home, feeling again the original light. This is an individual path of discovery where everyone has to play their part interrelating the tantric tissue of life during those times and situations that will bring you closer to the beginning.

Tantra emphasizes the couple in two opposite and complementary poles as the vibration between both engenders creative energy. When we use this potential force, we are able to illuminate more of our interior rooms.

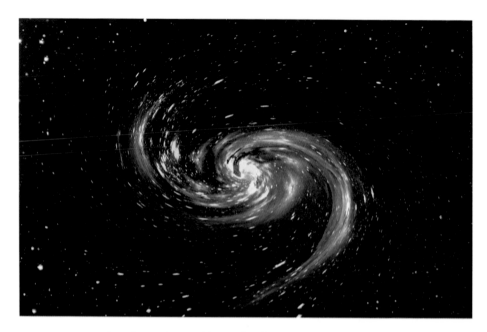

# Activating the chakras

The chakras are the existential molds of energy that connect and integrate us with all levels of existence. A chakra is an energy wheel of consciousness. Within each of us there is information so we can feel, perceive, think, create, act, experience, eat, drink, etc. When we suffer an emotional event, mental or not, the chakras may suffer or become blocked.

Our seven chakras are stairways that lift us away from the animal level into a higher level of spirituality. Daily, we pass from one plane to another. Tantra seeks to have all planes vibrate

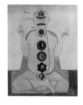

in harmony. In the same way a musician tests and tunes an instrument, a tantric takes care of the body, energy, and emotions so all the centers emit an adequate vibration.

The chakras are mostly activated through tantric sadhana, practices of the kriyas, or energy exercises that increase "spiritual vitamins" as each center begins to vibrate more and more and expands personal awareness.

In my other books (including *The Art of Tantra*), there are boxes with more detailed information about chakras.

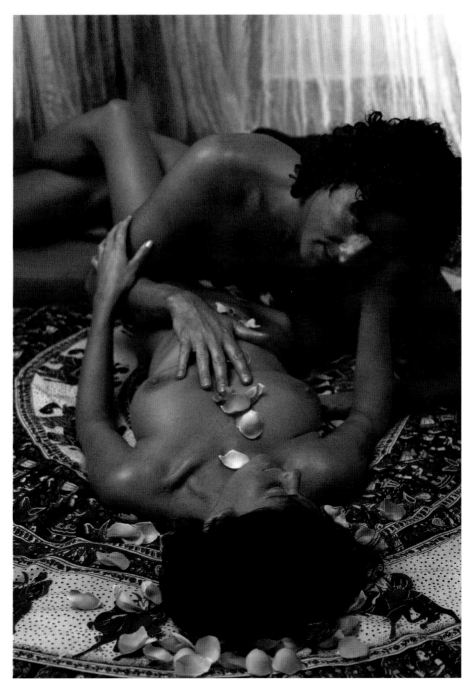

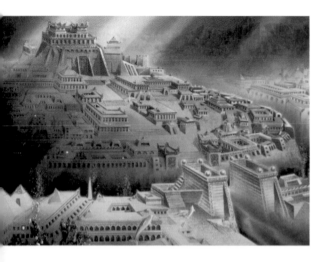

## Sexual energy: a human treasure

**Gourdjieff** and the Fourth Road.

Top illustration: the idealized Atlantis.

It is said that the women of Atlantis would nearly beg to receive a man's seed, his *bindu*, or ejaculation. In almost all cultures, people (Egyptian, Indian, Chinese, Druid, Atlantean, and Mayan, amongst others) have worshipped sexual energy and saw it as the raw material for spiritual transformation. The Gnostics refer to ejaculation as "internal alchemy"; Taoists speak of the Three Jewels; Gurdjieff mentions "*elioxhary*," meaning sperm. For Tantra, it is important not to waste semen nor sexual energy through excessive ejaculations (which is not the same as an orgasm), with either men or women.

Life gives us life, so we shouldn't waste it. Semen, or the bindu, has the potential to engender a new human being; it contains genetic information. If someone wants to become pregnant, the seed has to be planted in a spiritual land in order to open the path to the universe.

One may think, "Should I never ejaculate?" There are schools of thought that are more rigid about this, while others are more flexible. My suggestion, from personal experience and from the experiences of my students, is that you should ejaculate once for every 10 to 12 times you practice tantric sex; this allows you to conserve energy.

It is not advisable to start ejaculating during a crescent moon, as this will require more energy. Instead, you can do so during a full or waning moon. I still insist that the more you can hold off, the more this elixir will provide momentum, inspiration, enthusiasm, spiritual perception, and the desire to live and create.

This energy is developed through breathing techniques, mantras, meditations, learning, and the accumulation of prana in the chakras.

## Discover your individuality

"Individual" means "indivisible." When we do not feel fractioned, when we are full and complete, then we are individuals. Individuality is embodied by originality. Each person has a special gift, something that makes him or her unique. When an artist is highlighted, this happens through showing his or her originality and individuality.

Throughout history, individuals (who were the winners of the first race of 500 million sperm) have always worn (have shown its light) the qualities that the universe has given them.

In creation, there is individuality and diversity. One singer can give us a melody while another sings something different and both are exciting. In Tantra, our paths start in the same place because you cannot give what you do not have. First, we should be one, without divisions, without conflict, without disabling the psyche between good and bad or moral and immoral; we must be whole and should not set limits that do not actually exist.

When what we feel is in harmony with what we think, our actions will be balanced, harmonious. To the extent that the energy is increased by tantric practices featuring dances, massages, meditations, yoga, and sexual rites, we have a greater capacity for feeling closer to our individuality, **feeling like a drop ready to be dissolved in the sea.**

Paradoxically, we must first integrate our individuality, to discover

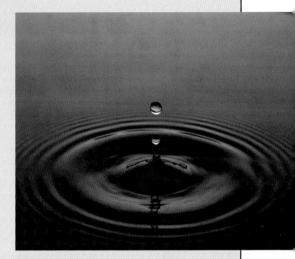

the light in order to disintegrate into the Supreme Light, for this is the purpose of life: lighting the human spirit with the divine.

When I was traveling in Mexico, one Shakti friend told me about the possible loneliness in feeling the "**age of the sun**," a necessary period to perceive our presence in harmony with the cosmic symphony. Certainly we need periods of solitude to generate fuel, to vibrate at our best. Through this, we will be ready to make a call to the other part, just like animals do. We attract what we emit, so these phases of our lives will raise and expand our individual light in order to meet with those to share our originality, love, and fusion, in which both disappear as individuals and integrate into the universal.

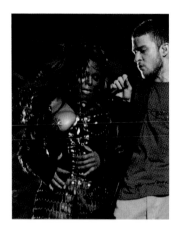
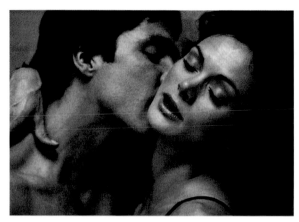

## Millennial sex secrets, today

While other countries were immersed in spiraling war and violence, American news went into alarm over the appearance of a female breast on television.

This work contains knowledge and, above all, practical exercises to learn to manage sexual energy. In ancient times, this knowledge was only known at the surface (although there has been a fight in every era of history...until today) and was found by spiritual seekers such as kings or Buddhas in pursuit of an inner awakening.

Religion and government spend too much time censoring sex. This topic is taboo in many regions of the globe (it is even today, after 10,000 years of supposed evolution). The prudish American society recoiled in fear from a popular singer's breast as if we had not all taken breast milk as our second food (the first food was the air). Is a breast not worthy of veneration? When your lover allows you to play with her breasts, is this not a course of pleasure? This raises the question, "Why do we condemn the female breast?"

When I was traveling through Mexico, I heard about the height of this repression in the plaza of La Diana in the Federal District. There is a statue of a nude woman that was ordered to wear clothes; how shameless, dressing a statue! Regardless, a 12-foot-high statue is in no danger of being violated.

There are many cases like this; there is an emphasis to censor everything that has to do with the naked body. It's as if there is a fear that society will overflow if it considers sex as something free.

What is the current status? When those who are children now reach adolescence, they will have witnessed thousands of violent images on television. TV news is infested with death and Machiavellian plans; films go even further! This is allowed but we censor scenes that show love and enjoyment; is this not completely absurd?

Regardless, thanks to the information we have available now, you can learn more than ever before about personal intimacy. Popular books such as *The Da Vinci Code* by Dan Brown, to name just one, are quite revealing of the historical and unnatural methods used by the church.

The Catholic Church is not the only institution that has condemned sex; almost all religions have gone to great lengths to hide valuable information. Organized religions, as you know, are no longer human. Tantra, on the other hand, is a reflection of wisdom and open to life itself. Life, among other things, is a phenomenon filled with sexual encounters.

# Did you know?

*There are many secrets that can be of good use to you:*

- Men can have orgasms without ejaculating.
- Women have a natural capacity to be multiorgasmic as a symbol to the goddess that connects us directly to the universe.
- Sexual energy is the key to climbing the ladder of spiritual evolution.
- Sexual repression is the fear of freedom.
- Sex is the highest spiritual manifestation on Earth: our duality yearns for originality.
- Breathing (air) and tantric sexual yoga techniques enliven sexual energy (fire).
- The attraction between the poles is inevitable.
- Sex is a source of creativity and the expansion of consciousness.
- Original sin (the first mistake) was to ejaculate ("that fruit you shall not eat, to only be fruitful and multiply"). The problem was not sex or nudity, but to ejaculate when there was no intention to procreate; this is when a man loses energy and decays the paradise that exists when individual consciousness is attached to the universal consciousness, a state of animal and weakness.

# Tantric objective

The main goal of Tantra is to enjoy life, to learn to play. In that game, we have to join the Principle Feminine (Shakti) and the Principle Masculine (Shiva) within us.

The first chakra is Shakti, represented by the kundalini energy. This coiled power should arouse and upload the main conduit, sushumna, and become one with Shiva (con-

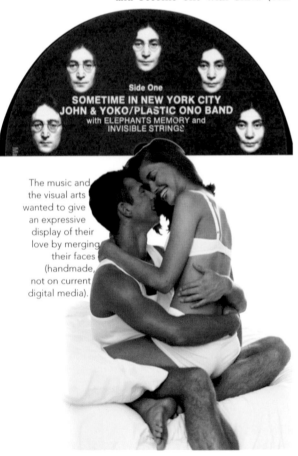

The music and the visual arts wanted to give an expressive display of their love by merging their faces (handmade, not on current digital media).

sciousness) at the top. This is the supreme tantric goal, to illuminate the consciousness, the cells, the soul . . . .

In order for this energy to wake and grow, you must perform the exercises and the sexual act to unite the energetic poles that generate the light.

From Jesus to Mary Magdalene to current followers of the Gnosis, everyone has had to perform a sexual initiation in order to illuminate the conscious. The energy of sex is a motor.

Use the form of conscious sexual energy in your favor. This is wise because the alternative is allowing your instinct's stronger awareness to make you its subject. Everything is connected. In order to channel and balance the sexual flow, it is necessary to tame the mind and breath. When we see sex as something natural, while remembering that it is esoteric and mystical, we are revealed to the deep end, the mystery of the game of the energies.

Whenever a tantric couple makes love, they know that it is in that moment that they have the ability to transcend their animal instincts and to enter the kingdom of light consciousness, pleasure, ecstasy, and the ability to stop time and therefore feel the spark of eternity that surrounds everything in every moment.

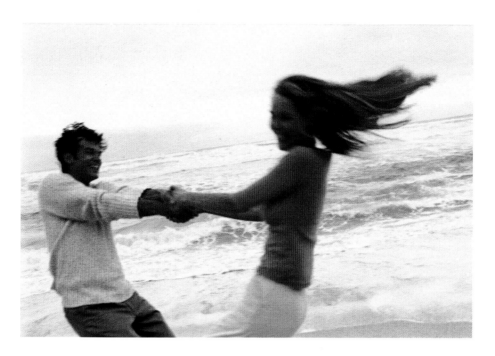

# Enjoy, live, celebrate, and transcend

And after the ritual? Tantra is an invitation to live as a king and queen, as co-creators of life, to become a Dionysius. When energy is well channeled, creativity arises: the desire to dance, to live, to laugh, to think, to drink good wine . . . a sense of wholeness appears, a connection with all of existence. This is a different approach to life. It is as if we had lived in black and white before Tantra, but now life has taken on new colors; the internal eye can capture new visions and can see reality clearly.

As it is not a religion, but a free way for sensitive, sensual, mystical, and creative people, it does not teach suffering or guilt; there is no cross to bear, or no seriousness—the most serious thing we can do is laugh. Tantra emphasizes joy, a celebration that each moment is a divine gift.

Nothing in Tantra is sacred or profane, since everything is within a sublime context. Everything is signed by the divine. As a mystic once said, "God is in all men, but not all men are in God, and that is why they suffer."

**Tantra is an invitation to live like a king and queen, as co-creators of life.**

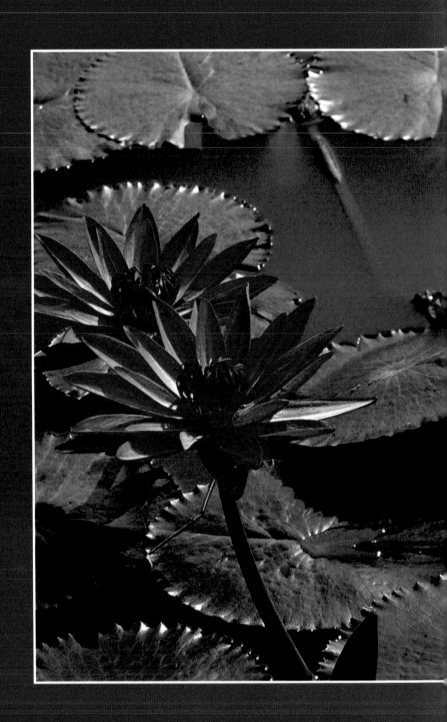

# Learning Tantra

"When the sleeping goddess Kundalini is awakened, through the grace of the teacher, all of the subtle lotuses and mundane bondages are pierced through and through. The wise person should rise willfully and firmly to the Goddess Kundalini, as it is she who gives miraculous powers to all."

*SHIVA SAMHITA*

The energy of Kundalini generates life in the human body.

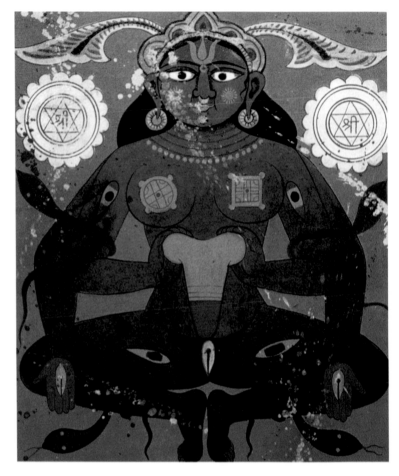

Imagination as mental energy is viewed by Tantra as a means to specify the physical plane as we imagine it.

# The use of sexual magic

Albert Einstein said that "imagination is more important than knowledge." When we imagine making magic, it is often used against us. Often, the imaginative energy ends up being in reality and generates conflict, unaware that there are laws of energy that span thought to action. Imagination and energy are viewed by Tantra as a means to narrow the physical plane of imagination. You always imagine first and then act (not counting instinctive actions). We must learn to use sexual magic to become stronger in life, love, and creativity. As a famous occultist said, "Sexual magic is the art and the science of achieving changes in consciousness according to the will."

Depending on the specific intention of what you want to achieve, different sexual magic is used: repetition of the mantras, a receptive and positive attitude, secret breathing techniques, energy accumulation, and visualizations.

"Magic" is derived from the Persian word magi, as in "teaching," "magician," "judge," "mogul," "magnificent," "master," magnanimous," and "magnetism." Even Alex took the name of The Great, derived from the Greek word mag: "large," "sublime," "and "magical."

Sexual energy can magically raise and magnetize the life of the Tantra practitioner.

# Kundalini: myths and realities

Kundalini energy creates life in the human body. We recieve, among other things, the masculine energy of the sun and the feminine energy of the Earth; the kundalini shakti energy is located on the first chakra and corresponds to female polarity, Shakti. On the other side, on the top of the head, is the male pole, consciousness, Shiva. In Tantra, the objective is the mystical encounter or marriage (union) of both energies.

*"When the sleeping goddess Kundalini is awakened by the grace of the Master, every subtle lotus and worldly attachments are transferred over and over again. The wise person should voluntarily and firmly rise to the goddess Kundalini as it is she who conferred all miraculous powers."*
SHIVA SAMHITA

To talk about the risks of prematurely awakening Kundalini would compare to the fear of hell that was infused in the Christian church. The human body must be prepared for a gradual rise in this energy. At its peak, it will increase enthusiasm, vitality, joy, consciousness, the state of love, creativity, and insight.

Tantra can be considered like a science experiment of consciousness. The disciple has to be true to himself, true to the practices, fully conscious, while at the same time flexible enough to adapt and to win the battle against laziness.

"Kundalini" literally means "coiled energy." Tantric exercises (including the act of sex) releases kundalini from sleep, and in doing so, a wild spark runs for miles through the skin, the blood, the chakras, and the source of new experience.

**Sexual magic is the art and science of occurring changes in the awareness in accordance with the will.**

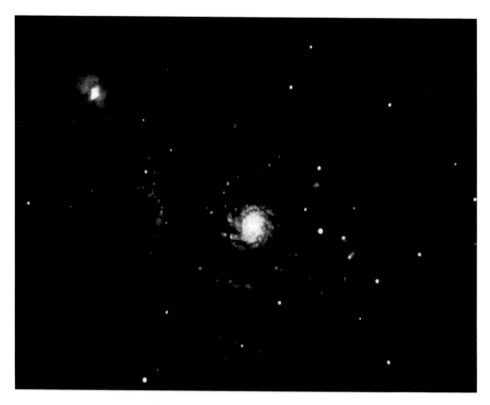

# Understanding the universe from a tantric perspective

**For Tantra, the Big Bang is a giant orgasmic explosion of light, creation, and awareness that generated the universe.**

Tantra does not ask why, but references what. It is an invitation for you to discover yourself and it offers actual techniqes. Tantra is a practical and experimental road; it does not focus solely on theory.

For Tantra, the Big Bang is a giant orgasmic explosion of light, creation, and awareness that generated the universe. Remember that the word "universe" means "a center." Just as the hub of a wheel is fixed, the circumference is what spins. The Universal Consciousness was created as a great Wheel of Life (Lilah). This game, in which everything revolves around the divine, is either perceived or not. This dance, the great cosmic movement of planets, galaxies, and solar systems, was created by Brahma, the creative function of the divine.

There are basic functions within the universe that result in daily life. Thus, there is a tantric trinity concerning their deities.

These aspects are much more related to our daily lives than we think. Do we not destroy things in our lives before creating something new? Does not the architect tear down old barns before building new ones? Do we not end one relationship while the door is open for a new one?

The destructive trinity, creation and conservation, is latent in the wave of life, only a matter of perceiving what aspects we regard and flowing with them. A tantric knows that everything is temporary.

## Trinity of tantric deities

1. **Brahma:** the role of Creation
2. **Shiva:** the role of Destruction
3. **Vishnu:** the role of Conservation

*These male deities have obvious female counterparts.*

1. **Saraswati:** consort of Brahma: wisdom, art, and creativity.
2. **Kali:** consort of Shiva: passion, sexual debauchery, and change.
3. **Lakshmi:** consort of Vishnu: tenderness, sweetness, and sublime love.

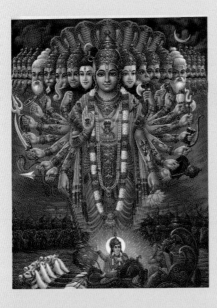 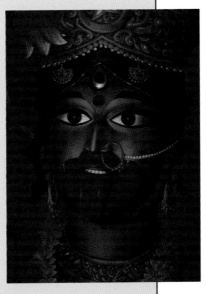

**Left image:**
Vishnu.

**Right image:**
The goddess Kali.

41

# 15 tantric exercises for couples

This is an invitation to explore new facets of your sexuality, sensuality, and seduction, to engender new sensations or sparks that can lead to a more profound fire. The motto is "playing with energy." There is no rush to enter the mind; this is a sequence that can make you feel the prolonged and awakening kundalini sexual energy in the moment. We will stimulate our senses from various angles.

## 1. THE NEW BIRTH

Lying in a fetal position with naked bodies, breathe slowly and deeply in unison to clear the mind. You must lay on your right side, opposite the heart. *Duration:* at least 10 minutes

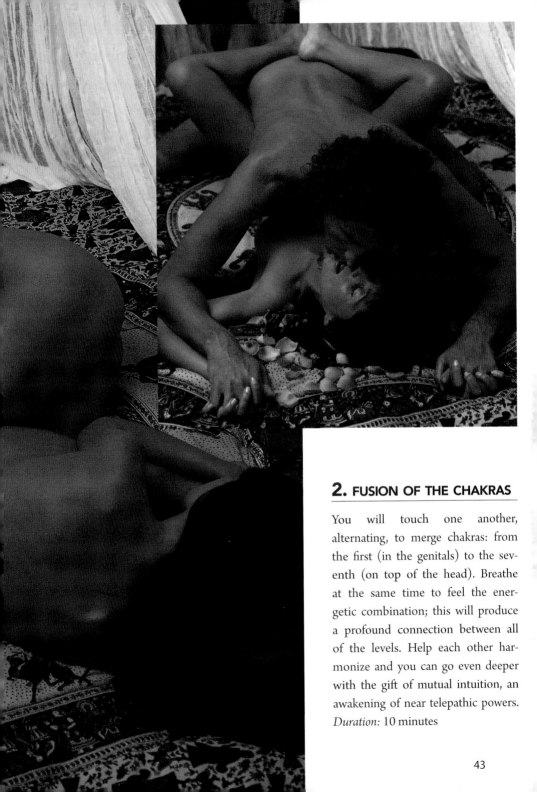

## 2. FUSION OF THE CHAKRAS

You will touch one another, alternating, to merge chakras: from the first (in the genitals) to the seventh (on top of the head). Breathe at the same time to feel the energetic combination; this will produce a profound connection between all of the levels. Help each other harmonize and you can go even deeper with the gift of mutual intuition, an awakening of near telepathic powers. *Duration:* 10 minutes

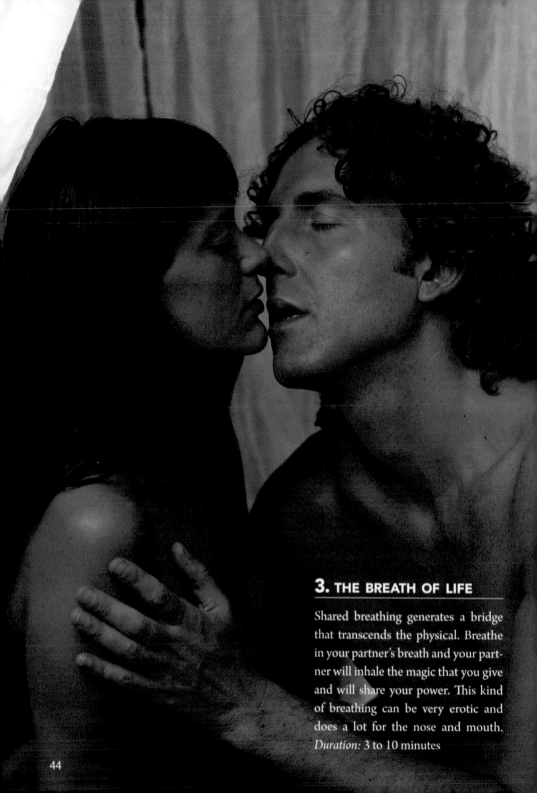

### 3. THE BREATH OF LIFE

Shared breathing generates a bridge that transcends the physical. Breathe in your partner's breath and your partner will inhale the magic that you give and will share your power. This kind of breathing can be very erotic and does a lot for the nose and mouth.
*Duration*: 3 to 10 minutes

## 4. THE TANTRIC EMBRACE

In Tantra, the embrace of Shiva and Shakti are synonymous. Let the sensations of attachment, fullness, and connection occur between both people. A hug can be a good preamble to having sex. The embrace of Shiva embraces the soul and fire; the embrace of Shakti embraces the moon, earth, and sea.
*Duration:* No time limit

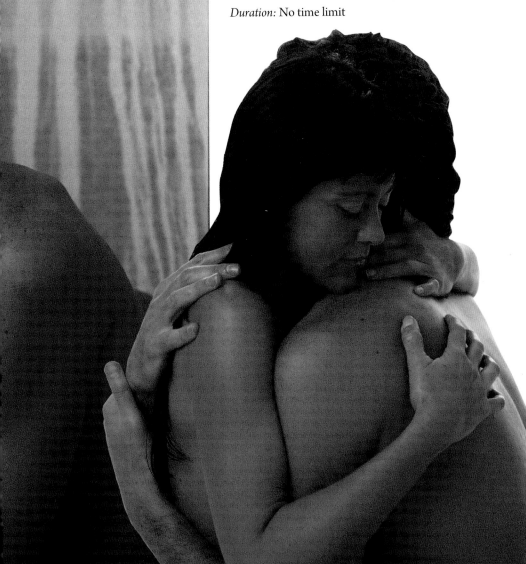

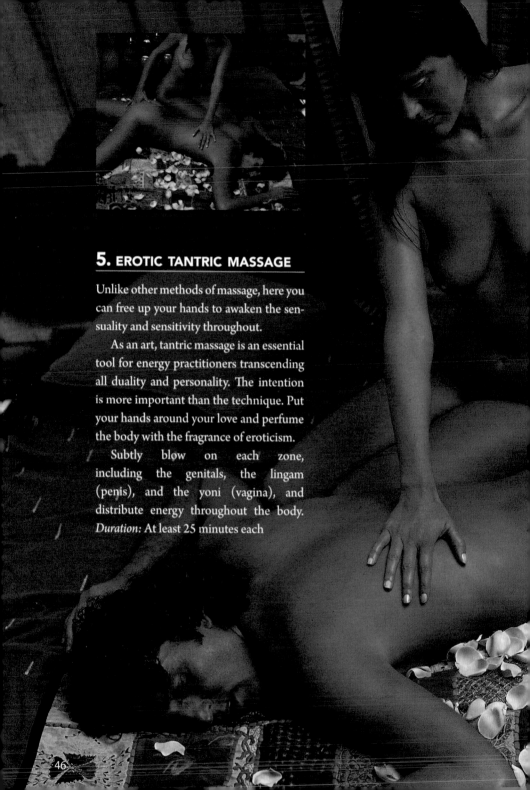

## 5. EROTIC TANTRIC MASSAGE

Unlike other methods of massage, here you can free up your hands to awaken the sensuality and sensitivity throughout.

As an art, tantric massage is an essential tool for energy practitioners transcending all duality and personality. The intention is more important than the technique. Put your hands around your love and perfume the body with the fragrance of eroticism.

Subtly blow on each zone, including the genitals, the lingam (penis), and the yoni (vagina), and distribute energy throughout the body. *Duration:* At least 25 minutes each

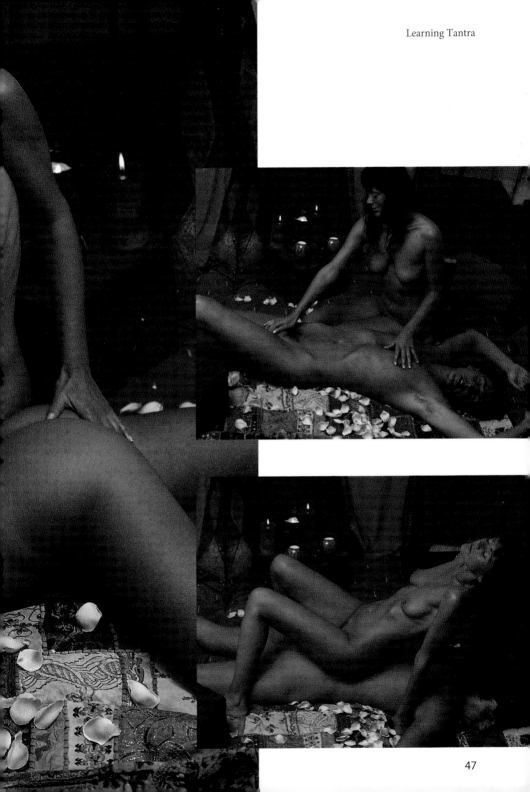

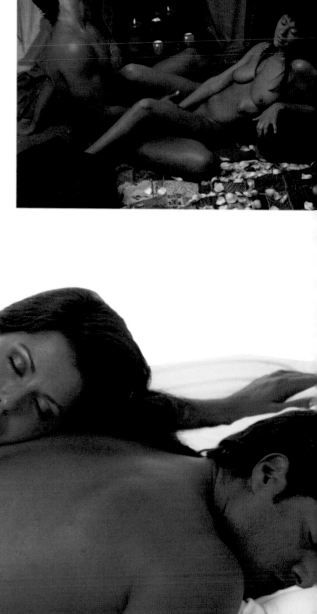

## 6. REST

Lying face down, align the chakras in a more subtle way; this will allow the mind to free all kinds of stress. Let the intoxicating sensations of being relaxed on both the inside and the outside extend to their total intensities. *Duration:* 5 to 15 minutes

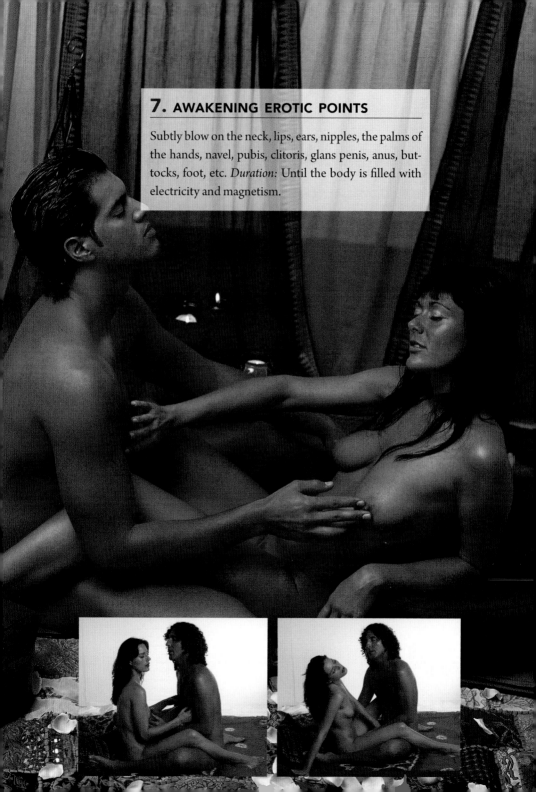

## 7. AWAKENING EROTIC POINTS

Subtly blow on the neck, lips, ears, nipples, the palms of the hands, navel, pubis, clitoris, glans penis, anus, buttocks, foot, etc. *Duration:* Until the body is filled with electricity and magnetism.

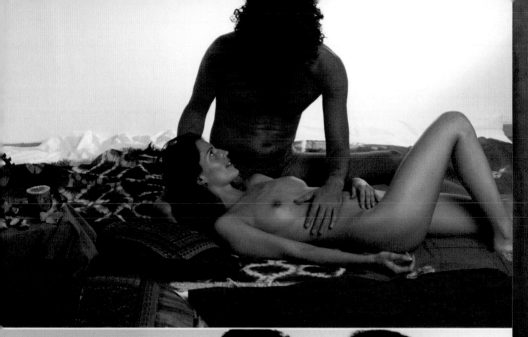

## 8. TOUCH AND AWARENESS

Softly touch your lover's body, with deep awareness, feeling their functions beyond the boundaries of the skin. Feel one another's hearts, stomachs, breathing, legs, hands, etc.

Touching is healing, a vehicle for expressing love and energy. *Duration:* 10 minutes

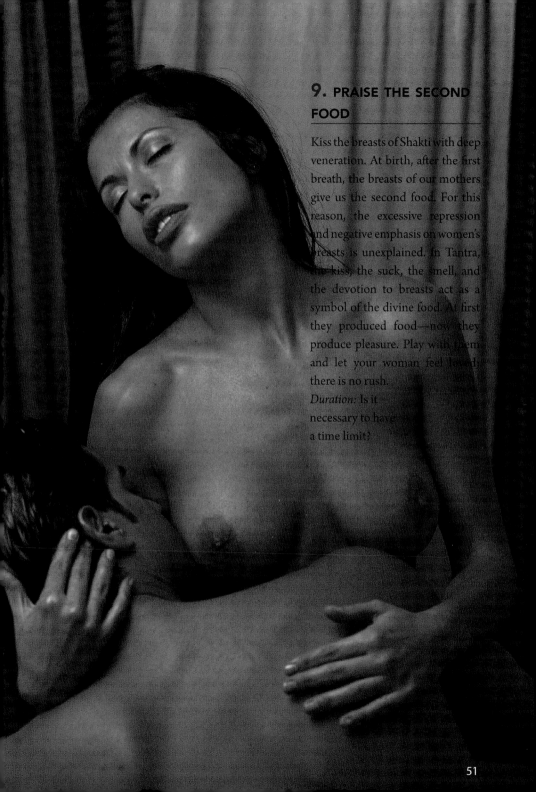

## 9. PRAISE THE SECOND FOOD

Kiss the breasts of Shakti with deep veneration. At birth, after the first breath, the breasts of our mothers give us the second food. For this reason, the excessive repression and negative emphasis on women's breasts is unexplained. In Tantra, the kiss, the suck, the smell, and the devotion to breasts act as a symbol of the divine food. At first they produced food—now they produce pleasure. Play with them and let your woman feel loved; there is no rush.

*Duration:* Is it necessary to have a time limit?

## 10. THE KISS OF THE BELOVED

Kiss softly and kiss deeply; bite, blow, connect tongues, etc. Kissing is an art within Tantra as well as a trigger for awakening sexual energy. When mouths and tongues are connected, sexual energy within the genitals is automatically awakened. This is because there is a meridian (nadi) of 72,000 points adorning the body from the tip of the tongue to the genitals. In the tantric texts, it states that one of the most erogenous zones of a woman's body is her upper lip.

Remember, the upper lip is connected to the clitoris through nadi energy.

Kissing the upper lip generates intense waves of pleasure throughout the body of Shakti. The *Kama Sutra* and *Ananga Ranga* also mention the importance of kissing the upper lip.

*Duration:* In general, this should not be excessive, as it can lead to premature ejaculation. The desire would be to alternate kisses so they increase the passion subtly.

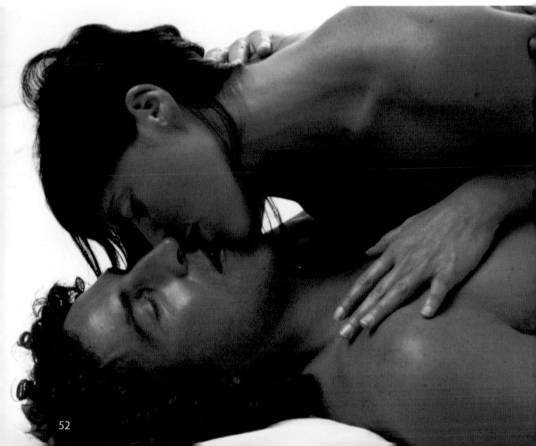

## 11. TOUCH AND EYE CONTACT

Play with touching each other and
deeply feel the essence
of eye contact.
Alternatively, let
the other person
see how you play
with your entire
body.
*Duration:* 10
minutes

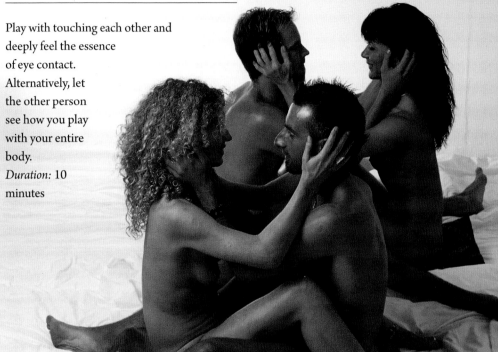

## 12. USING CRYSTALS AND STONES

The ancient Atlanteans kept information in
quartz. This is, in some ways, just like music
recorded on CDs. The stones contain life and
energy. Place all personal gems in your practice locations as opposed to highly magne-
tized areas. Leave your mind blank and
concentrate on superior strength; open
your third eye and concentrate on
the gem, focusing all of your power.
You can then carry it in your wallet
or clothes all day. *Duration:* 3
minutes

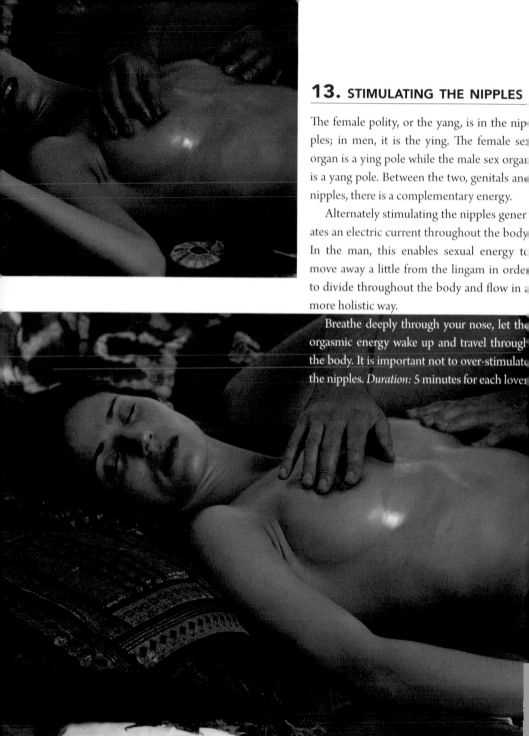

## 13. STIMULATING THE NIPPLES

The female polity, or the yang, is in the nipples; in men, it is the ying. The female sex organ is a ying pole while the male sex organ is a yang pole. Between the two, genitals and nipples, there is a complementary energy.

Alternately stimulating the nipples generates an electric current throughout the body. In the man, this enables sexual energy to move away a little from the lingam in order to divide throughout the body and flow in a more holistic way.

Breathe deeply through your nose, let the orgasmic energy wake up and travel through the body. It is important not to over-stimulate the nipples. *Duration:* 5 minutes for each lover.

## 14. BLINDFOLDS

We can remove the sense of sight in order to travel the interior world. While using a blindfold, slide a pen or your fingers across your lover's body. Make your lover feel your breath, your scent, and your presence. This is in invitation to take your lover through deep currents of pleasure. *Duration:* 10 minutes

## 15. YOUR CLOTHES ARE EXCITING

While clothing and accessories in the ancient art of Tantra are important, at the time there were no garters. Don't forget that we are gods. Some couples, however, are excited by costumes and Tantra does not rule out anything and always serves to turn on sexual power. You can play with sexy clothes to arouse desire. Suggest, provoke, and give a sexy dance; use your beloved seduction as a weapon to revolutionize your sexual energy. *Duration:* What you put on depends on what you want; prolong the excitement of your lover with your sensual movements.

For Tantra, to touch is to know. Touching and being touched brings down barriers, walls, and emotional defenses.

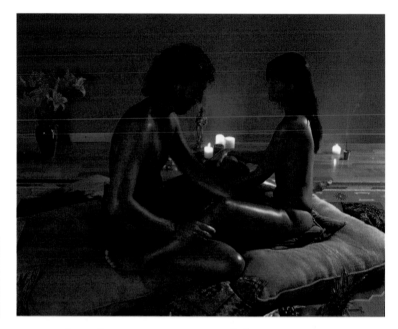

# Touch: the existential language

**Touch awakens, stimulates, energizes, and connects our senses while generating the feeling that we are not alone.**

In Tantra, to touch is to know. Touching and being touched brings down barriers, walls, and emotional defenses. In former times, people touched each other. Touch awakens, stimulates, energizes, and connects our senses while generating the feeling that we are not alone.

Studies on newborns, some cherished and some not, show tht the first group almost never cry, they smile, do not suffer from diseases, and are full of life. It is almost the opposite for the second group, those who do not receive the stimulus of touch.

Energy travels through the hands and arms as an extension of the heart. In tantric exercises, the stimulation of touch is almost always used. When you observe one tantric group of students touching each other with their naked bodies, you see a symphony of beauty, connection, sensuality, attraction, and delivery.

Sometimes there are those who, at first, feel rejection; their mental springs fire as if they saw something forbidden or sinful. I then stop them and ask, "What is normal? The war or the corruption? The fight or the unbridled competitiveness?

If you see two images, one of a group of people touching with

# The mystery of the five senses

The five senses are windows to the soul. Through physical senses, one can perceive and understand the world. In Tantra, we consciously encourage each of the senses to increase energy that in turn increases an internal sense, the sixth sense.

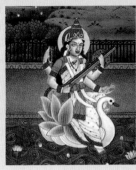

People say that women have an awakened sixth sense; this is true because women are more in touch with their perception while men are stuck in their heads (the venom of reason, control, and logic).

Each sense corresponds to a divinity. For example:

- Lakshmi: touch
- Kali: smell
- Vishnu: taste
- Saraswati: sound
- Brahma: view
- Shiva: internal sense

Remember that, to touch is to know; smell the perfume and activate the parts of the brain that deal with memory; please the feelings of desire and wake up to the kiss of vital energy; listen to the powers of imagination and be delighted by the sight of the beauty in the diversity of life; wake up and carry your inward energy in order to enhance your third eye, the clear, inner vision.

This is a time to arouse your *internal sense* by stimulating the five physical senses, a time to perceive rather than think. Perceiving establishes a direct connection to your intuitive wisdom (*prajna*) that connects us with universal wisdom.

**Energy travels through the hands and arms as extensions of the heart.**

sensuality, devotion, and lovingness, while the other is of a group planting bombs or committing murder—which is better?

We have become accustomed to watching too many movies with death and violence, but view naked bodies making love as something demonic. There are aspects of society that are unexplainable.

Remember: Tantra cures many mental viruses and silences the unnatural voices. This allows innocence and discovery to sprout in your life and to create a new body, a new universe of passion, sensations, and unity.

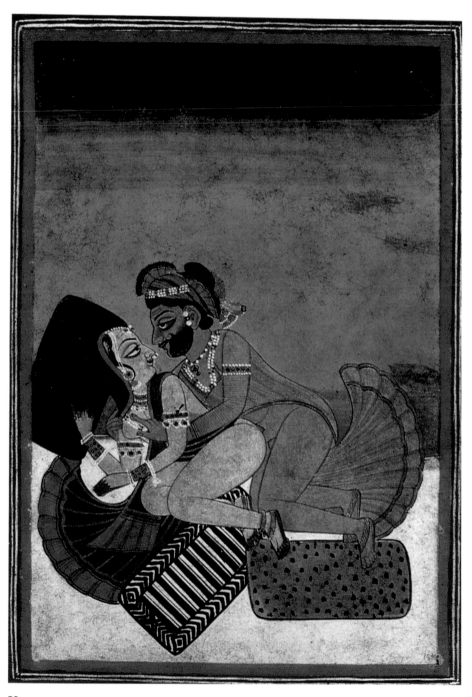

# Maithuna: the sexual rite of the five Ms

Tantra is a mystical invitation to explore the infinite dimensions of awareness through the act of sex. Improving one's sex life is just a natural consequence, but the real goal of these exercises is to fuse both poles in order to perceive the original unity.

There is a time of practice and experiential knowledge (which is the preamble to gaining this state) before you can swim in these ocean waters. Remember that maithuna is a sacred act of communion, pleasure, perception, awareness, attention, visualization, and a sea of feelings that open the heart, enliven the body and its functions, and detonate the expansion of consciousness.

The maithuna, known as the magical sexual act, involves special preparations. In my complementary book, *The Art of Tantra*, I explain step-by-step details, but in this work I go more into the ritual. To have a positive outcome with maithuna, attitude is the most important thing. If a partner does not vibrate in this frequency of high energy or treats it as something meaningless, the result will be a complete loss of energy and time for both parties.

In order for this sexual rite to be successful, it is advised to implement all, or at least part, of the following recommendations.

1. **Have an attitude that is consciously prepared** for a magical sexual encounter (you may want to prepare with a week of fasting to enhance sexual desires). Keep the chosen day in memory as something special in order to strengthen your spiritual consciousness.

2. **Decorate the room** with flowers, candles, cushions, sensual music, fabric, and anything that generates visual beauty, intimacy, and warmth. Place seven to nine candles in a circle. It is best if the predominant colors are red, orange, ocher, and violet.

3. **Reserve at least three to five hours** that won't be disturbed or interrupted.

4. **Prepare a few "festive" drinks** like a good champagne, wine, juices, or whatever you prefer. Enjoy the Five Ms (see the next page).

5. **Take a purifying shower.** Anoint the bodies with aromatic oils and give each other gentle massages in order to relax

Remember that maithuna is a sacred action of communion, pleasure, perception, awareness, attention, visualization, and a sea of feelings.

## The Five Ms

Mudra: cereals

Matsya: fish

Madya: wine

Mamsa: beef

Maithuna: sexual union

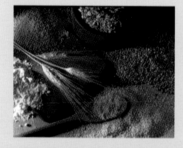

These elements represent the plant kingdom, the sea, the animal kingdom, and the divine existence.

**Cereals.** Earth: detachment from the terrestrial.

**Fish.** Water: mastery of breathing and emotions.

**Wine.** Fire: purification of the senses.

**Meat.** Air: understanding sounds.

**Maithuna (sexual union).** Space: mastery of desire and sexual energy.

your muscles. I also advise to do yoga stretches.

6. **Dance** freely for several minutes to sensual music or an intense drum.

7. **Make eye contact** for several minutes while sitting in a meditative pose. Smile. Be filled with tenderness and energy.

8. Perform lunar-solar alternative **breathing** by blocking one nostril and exhaling through the other; then do the reverse. Do this for about ten minutes.

9. Chant a **mantra**, perhaps with the help of a CD. For example, *Om bhur bwa swah* (the union of the three kingdoms); *Om mani padme hum* (Om: the union of lingam and yoni, or as another translation says, oh, the divine within me); *Om namah kundalini, Om namah Shiva, Om namah Shakti,* or *Om shakti hum.* All of these can be used to create an awareness of the sacred.

10. **Feel and honor** the male and female principles—Shakti in women and Shiva in men—with Pranava Mudra (hands on the chest, together).

11. **Share food.** Consciously eat a small part of each: wine, the elixir of the gods; meat, which represents the air; fish, the water of life; and

cereals and fruit, symbols of the land and its abundance. Meditate on this meaning. Do so slowly, near the sacred fire from firewood or simply candles.

12. **Stimulate the divine kundalini sexual energy** through the art of kissing and touching each other's bodies. Make contact with your tongues immediately after sex. Touch the entire body while emphasizing toes, hands and feet, navel, nipples, center of the chest, buttocks, crotch, armpits, shoulders, neck, lips, back, yoni, and lingam.

Apply, according to your preferences, scented oils or patchouli or sandalwood in all

areas; the body will be fragrant and delicious. Beforehand, make sure to allow the smell to recreate the natural odors of each.

13. **Visualize each other as Shiva and Shakti**, shedding your individual personalities completely.

14. Let **the wheel of love** begin to rotate freely. For example, practice oral sex, drinking Shakti's nectar like a precious pink fruit of eternal power, to practice penetrating the lingam gently. Allow your bodies to calmly try different postures of the *Kama Sutra*. Start with a slow and soft rhythm in order to arrive at a rising intensity. This rhythmic preamble

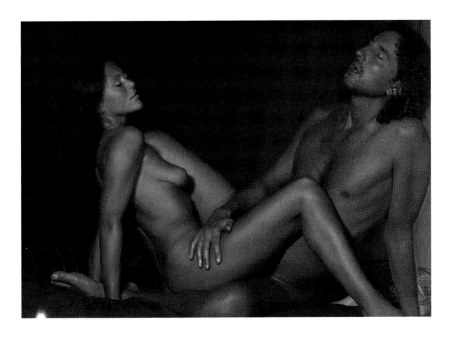

provides the energy to so as not to ejeculate prematurely. If Shiva gets too excited, the couple must stop. Practice these techniques to prevent ejaculation.

Women can access multiple orgasms any time they want. The couple can visualize something in this moment in order to concentrate on the extraordinary and magical power of the orgasm, language of the divine. Shiva will learn to transform the energy of ejaculation into a full-body orgasm, with waves of power and pleasure traveling through the entire body.

The longer the arrival of the orgasm is delayed, the deeper consciousness and sensation will be. The appearance of lights and sound within each one is normal, as it shows the elevation of potential sexual energy.

15. **Take a break every forty minutes;** meditate and connect your breathing in a *yab-yum* or "X" posture. With both legs open and lying face up, maintain the penetration and join hands. It is very beneficial at this point to recite a mantra together for several minutes.

The purpose of this phase is to open the mind's eye and distribute the energy and allow the meditation to go even deeper.

16. **Return to activating the energy** in order to promote a deeper point of consciousness. Travel through the emotional and spiritual world by the dance of love: the thirst of the Original One, Shiva and Shakti in fusion. You can try different tantric sex positions as you want to, allowing each to quench your desire without consuming it.

Finally, when you feel that the ritual is nearly over, meditate in deep communion, dance, eat, and celebrate the sparkle in the eyes, fire in the heart, and power in the entire body.

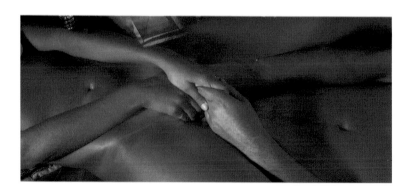

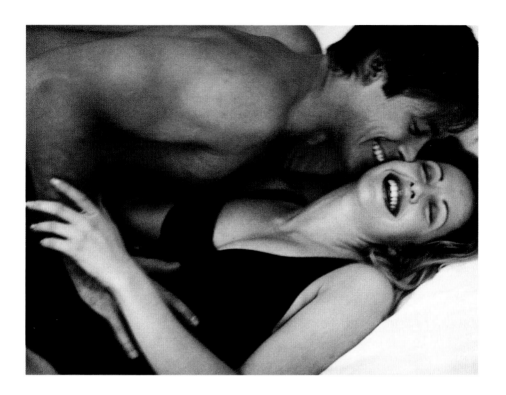

## Tantra in daily life

Tantra is more than a sexual rite with the power to transform ejaculation. That is only one chapter of the tantric book of life.

To apply Tantra is to live with **wealth**: creative, compassionate, and free thoughts, feelings, and acts. This is not only a supposed abundance of material goods, but rather is a way of seeing the world and living with beauty, art, wit, humor, love, and gentleness. Tantra is directed at all manifestations of life in order to enjoy everything without attachment or repression and to enjoy food, sex, travel, silence, dance, caresses, work, and relationships.

In my new project, *El Tao del Tantra*, I start with an essay on the style of tantric life, how to read the signs that allow us to realize that we're living a full life and enjoying the most out of our existence.

Tantra applies to your life like all art, knowing what you need, what you want, and what you desire to create.

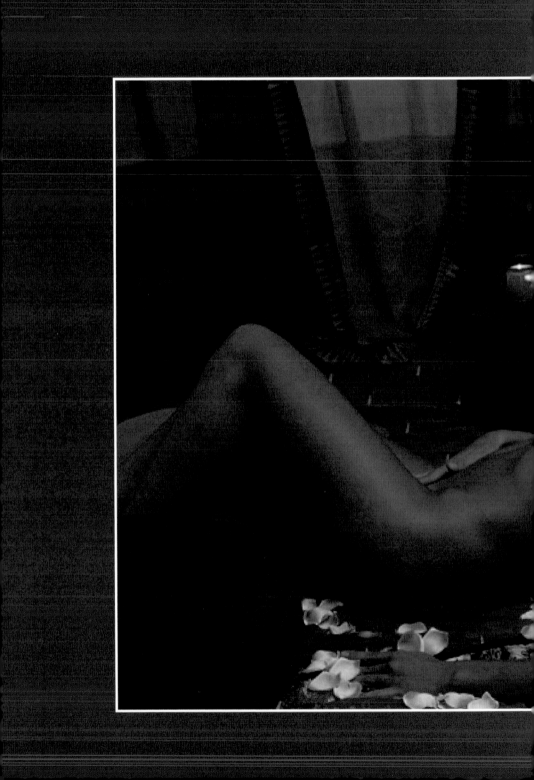

# The tantric woman

*"How delightful an instrument is woman when touched; capable of producing more exquisite harmonies or executing the most complicated variations of love and of giving the most divine of erotic pleasures."*

ANANGA RANGA

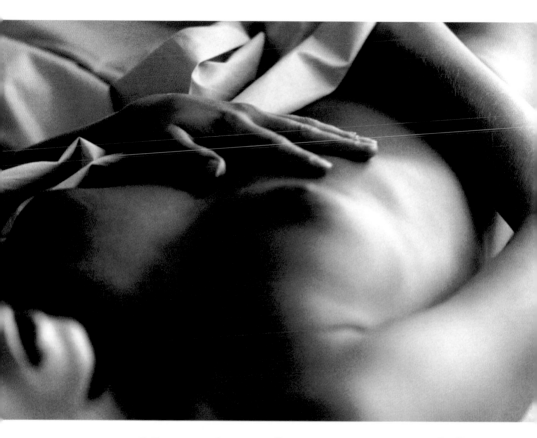

# Knowing the inner goddess

*"Oh, devotee! If you aspire to paradise, look to where the women of lust dwell."*
KUTTNI MAHATMYAM

Even the most submissive woman is internally engraved with the stigma of the goddess. During the centuries of patriarchal culture, there was an emphasis on censoring the divine feminine energy. Goddess worship goes all the way back to the beginning. Over 9,000 years ago, clans were ruled by a goddess; they were matriarchal societies. Men hunted and women farmed the land and raised the children, but it was the female criteria that governed the standards of life.

During the times of little hunting, men also cultivated the land and pastored the sheep, which was not to his liking. This is when the first revolts began. In the novel *El Secreto de la Diosa (The Secret of the Goddess)*, this is all relayed, with excitement. Moreover, men did not know that they were also the cause of childbirth. They believed that women invoked the goddess of fertility and were unaware that it came from the union of an egg with sperm. When men started to discover this, there came the second rebellion, strong and violent, that crushed female power.

Throughout history, men have been prevalent in the detriment of women, seeking to silence them.

In reality, just look at the covers of major magazines; virtually every one of them reflects feminine beauty. In Tantra, there is a special emphasis placed on women and the exquisite feminine values.

The laws of the universe contain laws of balance. Shakti and Shiva are eternally complementary; their opposite energies reflect permanent attraction. Life is made of this same attraction of the poles. The light surges through the connection of the two polarities. Similar poles create a short circuit; opposite poles generate light.

Therefore, Shakti is a complementary energy that is equally as important as Shiva. Energy and consciousness work together in harmony.

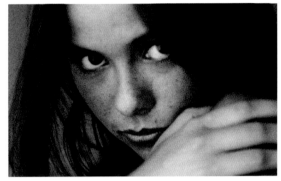

To know and feel Shakti (the goddess), or rather, to "feel and then know" (the tantric formula), it's important to silence the personality because divinity is the voice of essense. The personality, or the ego, with its imperfections, weaknesses, and shadows, cannot begin to fully perceive the goddess.

Within the essence of every man and every woman vibrates the divinity, in the core of their beings. Dances, meditation, raising energy, rituals, mantras, and sexual exercises are the tantric tools to awaken the goddess.

The classic Tantra text *Candamaharosana* says, "The Woman is the initiator, the procreative, the evocative delight of the Three Worlds, kind and compassionate. Like the object of the five senses, woman is blessed with the divine form."

Shakti is pure sexual energy: sensuality, perception, receptivity, and sensitivity. It is adhered with fire to the skin of every woman.

With only a single look, the woman can enchant and seduce.

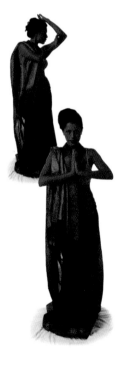

# Discover your multiorgasmic capacity

*"The ordinary sexual orgasm looks like madness. Tantric orgasm is a relaxed and deep meditation. You can gratify everything you want because you will not lose energy, but will increase it. Just find the opposite pole and your energy is renewed. The act of tantric love can be done as many times as you want . . . and the ecstasy will last hours, even days. It depends on how deeply you have surrendered yourself to him. With the tantric orgasm experience, you feel relaxed, calm, at home, without violence, without anger, and without depression for entire days."*

OSHO

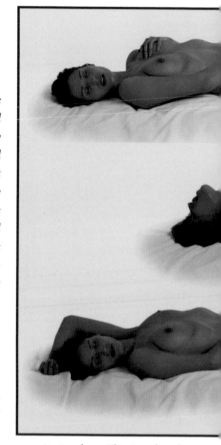

Throughout history, many women have been mutilate and have had their sexual expressions censored. Currently, however, there is a new force of female energy that is empowering women. This is a new and liberating awakening that seeks to find greater fulfillment in life. Although many women still suffer from the heavy yoke of submission and dependence, there is a great world movement of yin energy everywhere.

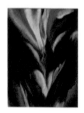

Every woman has the ability to reach multiple orgasms naturally. But each personal story finds that, for one reason or another, this

capacity is asleep. This is either due to repression in childhood, because of a castrating father or husband, from shame, because of unnatural ideas of sin, or physical problems; for these reasons, women turn away from this natural gift—the connection with the divine through orgasm.

The divine will visit, but first you have to accept your body. The female body is poetry in action, and always remember that all woman, all, have their own charm and are

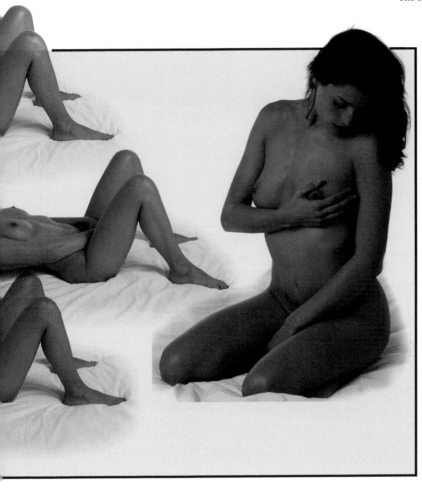

Every woman has a capacity, touch, and personal stamp that makes her different; your honey does not have the same taste as another.

attractive. Feel that you are unique and that there is no one like you in the universe: every woman has a capacity, touch, and personal stamp that make her different; your honey does not have the same taste as another.

What is it that makes divas (from Sanskrit deva "minor goddess") Sophia Loren, Angelina Jolie, Monica Bellucci, Nicole Kidman, or Penelope Cruz have an aura of light, magnetic attraction, "Cleopatra" to others? Because they emit a special energy, a strong charm, an awakened feminine spell. This is why women are not mentioned in religion, because men would lose power!

It has been shown (by various studies and practices) that, apart from any other circumstance, many

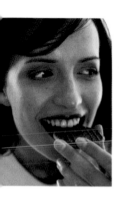

women have not known what an orgasm is.

Moreover, the Shaktis multiorgasmics that I've met strongly claim that this is an electrifying feeling distributed throughout the body. It has its trigger in the sexual area and its mouth and implosion zone in the brain so that energy flows throughout the spinal column . . . the tantric journey!

I sympathize with them; one becomes like a receptacle where God visits you; you dive into an unsurpassed ecstasy. The power that women transmit through an orgasm to herself, to the man, and to the entire universe is the **power of creation**.

## Unleash your power

Being one is actually a flooding of the consciousness, your body, and psyche with orgasmic energy. First, you must accept your body. Rub it with aromatic oils, touch yourself, dance alone or naked with a friend in a free and unrestrained manner to tribal music while repeatedly moving your hips and making sounds to awaken your erogenous zones. You must forgive your parents, husbands, lovers, and priests (they didn't know that they were suppressing you).

Breathe deeply with these practices while you stimulate your

Feel as if you're Aphrodite, change your hairstyle, and enjoy food (especially chocolate).

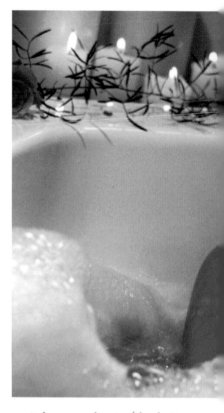

genitals, your clitoris (the button that awakens the divinity in you); practice yoga, take a bath in the tub, dress as you really are (a goddess), feel as if you're Aphrodite, change your hairstyle, and enjoy food (especially chocolate). In short, free yourself! Do not make obstacles for yourself and if this fails, you can find a new lover . . . a better lover.

Let that new energy gradually enhance itself inside of you. Avoid any notion of false mortality and be guided by the voice of your heart

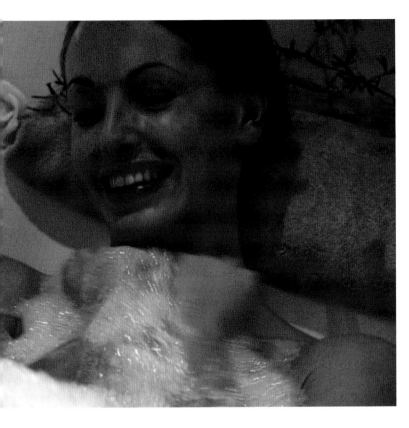

Practice yoga, take full baths, and dress like what you really are: a goddess

as was previously done by the former priestesses and initiators of the mysteries of sex.

## Realize your fantasies

I remember a young patient who consulted me in my work as a life coach. Despite feeling pretty, for various reasons, she felt submerged in the swamp of anorgasmia. We started to work and investigated several aspects that had been neglected and others that were missing.

Amongst other things, I had her write erotic fantasies, her deepest desires as if I could make them a reality in her psyche. She wrote more erotic stories, both intense and adventurous; what a different life she led in these stories! I explained that if we actually allow ourselves to experience desire, we can grow and evolve, and we can finally find satisfaction. As if it were too strict and puritanical, I suggested that we put an ad in the paper as if she were

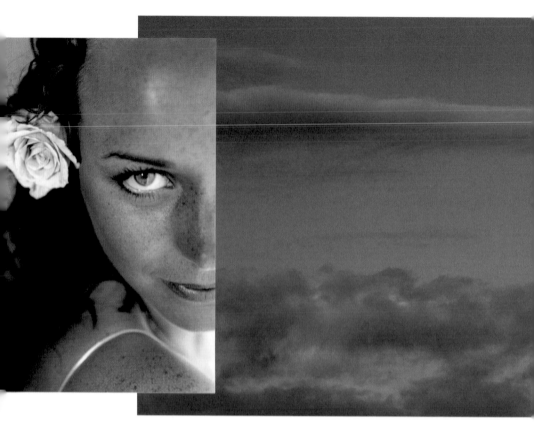

offering sexual services. She made quite the face! While she didn't actually offer any sexual services, it was important that she heard the voice messages left by men; it was what she needed to hear. Even though not everyone was a poet, this helped show that words have the power to move mountains and in this case, unlock the doors to the sleeping goddess waiting inside.

## Other approaches

Less than one hundred years ago, Sigmund Freud made a distinction between the clitoral and vaginal orgasm. He was completely unaware that, for 5,000 years, Tantra did not generate any divisions or theorize too much, but simply experienced. The tantric orgasm, or multiple-wave Happiness, is a mega-orgasm. It can last between 10 and 20 minutes and women can have up to sixty orgasms in "a normal day!"

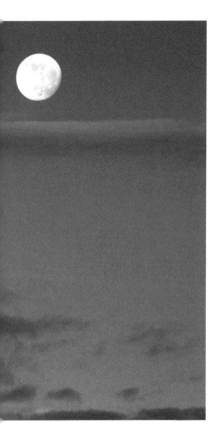

release body rigidity and conflicts that produced increased releases and energy that could enhance orgasmic waves. According to Reich, who had just freed his own sexuality, one may experience the full potential in life via these orgasms. Tantra says the same.

Tantra calls the clitoris the "jewel in the crown" and the G-spot the "secret treasure." Both should be stimulated in order to access multiple orgasms.

In his book *Exploring the Hidden Power of Female Sexuality*, Maitreyi D. Piontek says that "Many women live their entire lives without experiencing an orgasm and have a feeling of missing out. Others suffer for not being able to live it. Some women need it daily while others, as the American ex-prostitute Anne Sprinkle, talk about mega-orgasms, which last about fifteen minutes. She claims she needs to have one every couple of months to maintain her well-being.

Wilhelm Reich called this phenomenon a "Power Orgasm" and unveiled a series of exercises to

## Recognize a real orgasm

A man can find out if his partner is having a real orgasm by placing a finger in the anal area. If it contracts repeatedly, opening and closing, the orgasm is real. The women who just scream, cry, and kick . . . are only faking it.

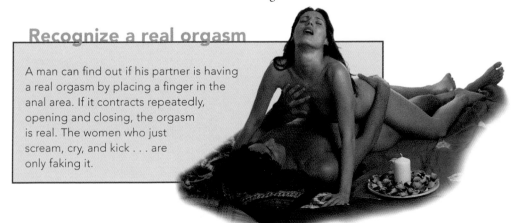

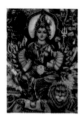

The goddess Shakti is pure sexual energy and is manifested in every woman.

Many women experience orgasms when masturbating or being touched by their partners, but not during intercourse. Others live spiritual experiences during the relationship. As we can see, the female orgasm is experienced and valued in very particular ways."

Female sexuality works best if you have the mind, body, chakras, and sexual doors open like a flower.

## The potency of your feminine power

Remember, feel it: in your uterus is a legacy, a stigma, a strong source of life. A life is reflected within you; you can generate a new being, both physical and spiritual. As a woman, you are an energetic embryo, a dynamo, a crucible, a treasure of light.

Be aware that you are one with the moon, the sea, the earth, nature, and with all female principles. Breathe them in, convert them into a meditation. You are the night, stars, flowers, and the mystique of life. Join that with power; it is yours, you belong.

In my seminars about Tantra for women they feel a magical power, a communion, and a very powerful aura of charm that binds ritual Shaktis, both physical and spiritual. And although I am not a woman, I can feel Shakti in me, complementing the primary androgyne through sensuality, responsiveness, and sensitivity, so that I do not lose my male power, but on the contrary, they complement each other.

Female power is expansive and as deep as the ocean, but also domestic and devotional. In the cults of antiquity there were rituals among women, naked, worshiping fire and the forces of nature. The contemporary woman has to append to her personal care a sense of *glamor* and independence, as well as the mystical and mysteries that save each heart.

For example, in traditional Eastern cultures, when a Shakti was expecting a child, she would meet with other women to dance and sing at the arrival of their offspring. The mother gave birth during the dance! Or she went to the river at the time of birth, poked a stick in the water while holding strongly with one hand and collecting the newborn with the other. Who could deny that huge power?

The intelligent and sensual contemporary woman knows that in herself there is an engine flowing through the veins and mutters a sense of life in her ear: "You are a goddess; wake up, enjoy, celebrate, sing the eternal song of praise to the divine."

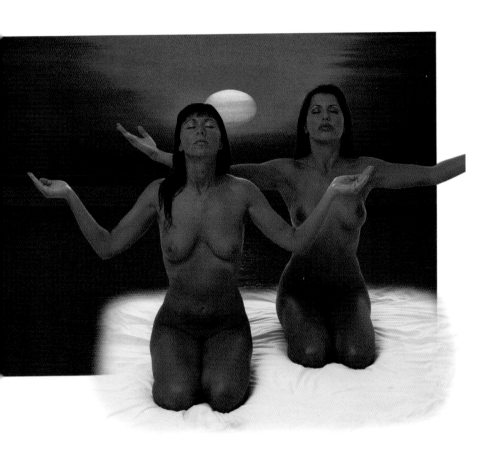

## Shakti and enchantment

The sensation felt by placing your head in the lap and breasts of a woman and relaxing while she caresses your hair is one of the more immersive experiences on this planet.

When a woman, in addition to her natural eroticism, uses her sweetness, her eyes, and the soft tone of her voice to open all doors. In ancient India, it was considered normal when two women had intimate relationships between each other. And it's not surprising, giving the complicity between women, that they can perfectly understand their secret language.

Physical contact between women has always been viewed as normal and even healthy in Eastern cultures.

**In the ancient cults, there were rituals between women, naked, worshiping fire and the forces of nature**

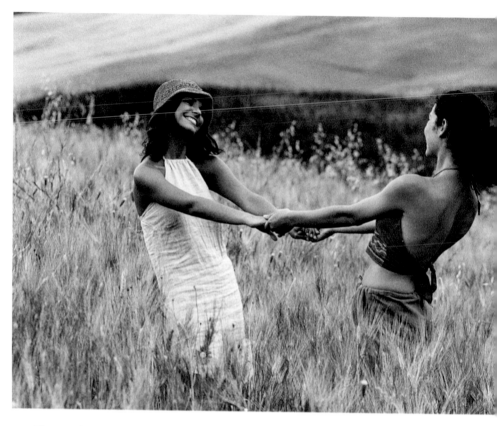

**The real encounter is of woman with woman, where neither of the two takes on the role of the male.**

More than 9,000 years ago, women lived together and slept in the same bed, were lovers and friends, and these relationships were not prevented by men. Even the *Ramayana*, the classic text of India, says, ". . . there were countless women passed out on carpets after spending the night playing sensual games. Their breath smelled of subtly sweet wine. Some smelled each other's lips while dreaming as if they were the lips of their owners. Their passion-ate arousal forced these beautiful sleeping girls to have sex with their companions. Some slept with their rich robes and adorned bracelets; others were laid about their peers on each other's bellies, breasts, thighs, or backs while hugging affection-ately with arms entwined. Women with slender waists laid together in their sweet, intoxicating dreams."

The *Kama Sutra* mentions women who were mutually satisfied; it also paints Krishna with his 108

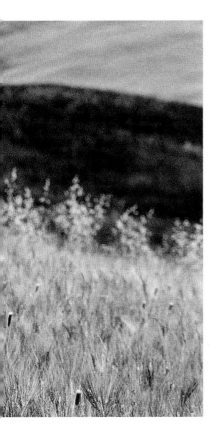

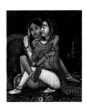

Tantra moves to awaken the nature of Kundalini Shakti in every woman. Without mental conflicts, as a sacred game of preparation to receive Shiva.

## Two women

Throughout history, many women have been openly in love with other women, as in the case of writer Virginia Woolf or the painter Frida Kahlo. In books such as *De Mujer a Mujer (Woman to Woman)*, by Monica Campos, letters were published between women who were known to have lived the most passionate romances.

Today it has been found that Europe grows in the number of women who are attracted to other women, awakening their natural androgynous energy, without meaning that they need to become male. The real encounter is of female and female, where neither takes the role of the male.

Tantra moves to awaken the nature of *Kundalini Shakti* in every woman—without mental conflicts, as a sacred game of preparation to receive Shiva. The female yin energy, in opposition of the male yang, is absorbing, nourishing, perceptual, permeable, and able to accept the same energy in order to expand and nourish each other. Yin energy can excite and raise the same yin energy. Shakti with Shakti means ignition. But as with electricity, masculine power is needed to ignite a light.

*gopis* (sensual women), illustrating the general sweet playing amongst them. While sexual union is not the main topic among women, throughout history the essence of yin with yin has been present. In the cultures of India, Egypt, Africa, Asia, the Pacific Islands, South America, and the East, the sensual relationship between women was seen as something beautiful, devoid of lust and perversion. On the contrary, it was seen as life playing with life.

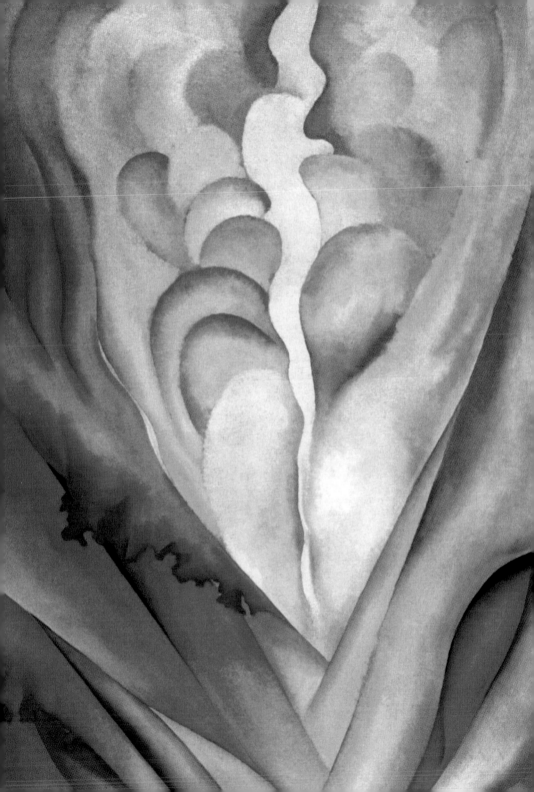

# Erotic points of the female body

Interestingly, not only are many women ignorant about their own bodies, but many don't even know where the G-spot is located. The problem is the lack of education both in school and in the family, or the fact that certain issues are considered taboo, preventing the discovery of the fantastic universe that is the human body.

Knowing the anatomy itself is basic to the awakening of Eros, the erotic and spiritual energy. This sacred fire, which is the sexual energy, is ignited by the stimulation of areas with the greatest sensitivity. These areas react to a certain rhythm, touch, visual stimuli, physical posture, and even dance. I have been surprised to find, in various seminars, that some Shaktis can have orgasms from dancing and tantric breathing. The vital energy responds to the call of fulfillment and is a manifestation of the inner goddess.

The points are many and varied; I have summarized more information in the following pages. There are also many different ways to stimulate them. For example, we know that many people have been excited by the jet from the end of the shower hose. Every person's body is sensitive to different stimuli. Tantra recommends stimulating the neck, mouth, ears, armpits, chest, nipples, hands, navel, pubis, clitoris, G-spot, buttocks, anus, crotch, and even the toes. Take time for yourself without interruption and increase your own pleasure while discovering every corner of your body, loving it while filling it with pleasure, communion, and joy. Place rose oil, jasmine, sandalwood, patchouli, musk or more delicate aromas as you prefer and unite each part to feel everything as a single unit.

**Not only are many women ignorant about their own bodies, but many don't even know where the G-spot is located.**

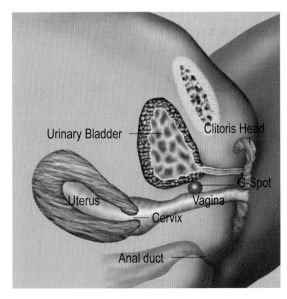

79

# Electricity and energy

When you exercise tantric practices, your entire body is electrified with dynamism, light, and vitality, and a strong vibration surrounds you; and this is not to mention the esoteric side.

The phrase **"full of light"** is not a poetic phrase, but a reality. When oxygen and prana fill the cells with light, organs are nourished, the heart and brain's functions are improved, and the potential sexual Kundalini energy is increased.

By increasing your vibration, you start to connect with other vibrational levels of existence which wil furnish experiences that create chords to that vibration. If you vibrate in a bright state, illuminated, circumstances will be favorable for your destiny to be fulfilled.

Some students, after some time, call me surprised because a pending business issue has been solved at last. A pending project or environment and atmosphere of your home changes. Tantra creates a **special alchemy with energy**, the transformation of polarity.

The tantric energy produces reconciliation, magnetism, and enchantment . . . but you have to **practice**. Forget being lazy; prepare

**If you vibrate in a bright state, illuminated, circumstances will be favorable for your destiny to be fulfilled.**

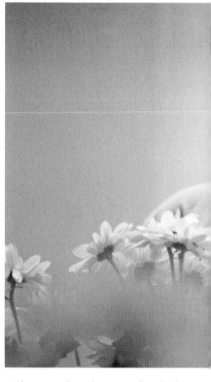

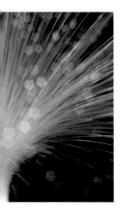

with yoga, breathing, and a little bit of physical activity. You have to remove **your own energetic treasure**; otherwise your life will be in black and white and not in color.

Have you heard of **pheromones**? This is the sexual fragrance that everyone has and everyone smells when we feel attracted or when we attract someone. This personal scent is a powerful aphrodisiac. Very small molecules control behavior and sexual attraction. Pheromones are transmitted through the skin and are often found in body fluids.

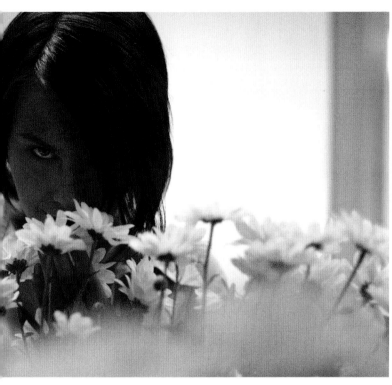

**Personal odor is a powerful aphrodisiac.**

In Japan (and now in other countries), it is possible to buy used women's underwear; anyone willing to pay the exorbitant sums of money required can recreate the intimate scent of a woman. This is just one example of how body odor is a powerful source of attraction; we should not hide such a powerful and natural aphrodisiac.

Previously, there were similar cases to that of Napoleon, who wouldn't wash after making love with Josephine so he could continue to feel her body odor. But hygiene is essential in Tantra, without taking away the powerful seduction of pheromones.

A tantric seeks to stimulate energy through each channel (*nostrils*) through which the **prana** (energy) will electrify "rivers of living water." No wonder the slogan is none other than to extend personal aura and consciousness into a much deeper state with evolutionary, bright, and energetic realities.

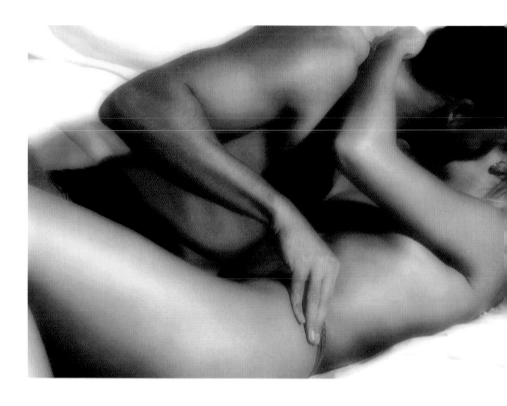

# The rhythm of Shakti

Women respond to a slower and more prolonged sexual stimulation. At the start of contact, many women can feel closed, blocked, or timid. But once you get to the physical heat, the energy, and the electric current and magnetism of somewhere else, every barrier falls and the entire mask is removed and the nakedness of this energy is presented as a fire.

When a woman is aroused, a dynamic vitality takes over and ignites the heart, genitals, and skin of Shakti. Shiva must understand that Shakti needs to be stimulated; once lit, man must become essentially passive in order to allow the increasing flood of Shakti to be released.

By stimulating erotic parts of a woman's body, the kundalini awakens and moves like a flame of fire. It is important for Shakti to guide your energy towards the top of your head, your spiritual zone, through visualizations, mantras, and breathing.

# The three types of yoni

In the famous texts the *Kama Sutra* and the *Anaga Ranga*, female sexual organs are classified into three basic types shown below.

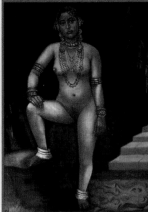

## The Stag

This yoni does not exceed 12 cm deep and is considered the small dimension.

The body of this woman is rather immature, infantile, like of an adolescent, smooth and shapely, with large breasts and strong hips. These women have active minds and their yoni juice is a delicious perfume like a flower. They feed moderately and love making love at any hour.

## The Mare

This yoni is around 18 cm deep and is considered the middle. The bodies of these women are subtle with medium-sized breasts, wide hips, and a rather bulky stomach. They have beautiful and harmonious hands and feet, long necks, and sunken foreheads. These women have big eyes and mouths and require a slow pace to achieve orgasm.

## The Elephant

This yoni is about 25 cm deep and is considered a large dimension. The Shaktis are busy and insatiable when it comes to making love. Their faces are wide and their voices are hard and rough. They eat loudly and their limbs are usually short. These women's secretions emanate a strong odor.

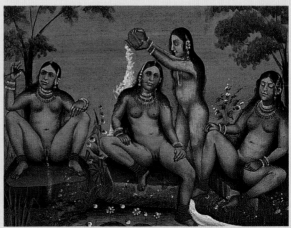

# The erogenous zones of women

Many women suffer from anorgasmia, the lack of orgasms, but not without excitement or pleasure. The causes can be varied, but rarely have to do with physical or organic matter. We must look for other reasons: anxiety, taboos, prejudices, fears, guilt, lack of communication, inhibition, or, of course, inadequate stimulation by their partner.

The woman must give herself to sex without fear or guilt of any kind, carried away by her feelings while knowing that pleasure does not have to be limited to the genital areas. In fact, the biggest human sex organ is the skin. On it, some parts are especially sensitive because there are nerve endings that react to any stimulus (fondling, kissing, nibbling, pressure, friction). These are the erogenous zones. In reality, a woman's entire body is erogenous if there are no barriers.

**Playing with her hair** allows various sensations of pleasure: slip your fingers through her hair from the root to the tip. As a massage, this is very pleasant.

Without taking time to stop, we have **the neck**, the entry to intimacy. This is one of the most erogenous zones of the female body. Your back, neck, behind the ears . . . the entire body is an area worth exploring. Make sure to be calm and careful as women can dip into waves of excitement.

**Lips** are one of the most sensitive areas of the body, where we kiss, the first sign of attraction.

It is extremely stimulating for couples to kiss slowly and gently, alternating the upper and lower lips or the tip of the tongue.

Slowly moving away from the neck, softly work towards the **back**, barely touching the skin with your fingertips, lips, or even nails. On her back, the most sensitive areas are between the shoulder blades and lower back and at the top of the buttocks. There is also a special point around the **sacrum** that you can press gently.

**Breasts** are one of the most erogenous zones of women, especially the nipples. The carressing should not come directly on the nipples, but should start with the part of the breast closest to the armpit with circular friction. Her nipples will quickly notice the excitement and will do so more if they are touched with fingers or lips. When they are erect, a puff of air on them will increase the pleasure.

The **navel** is an area that is often overlooked and is highly sensitive, especially if stimulated with an "aid" such as a cherry or strawberry. The navel is a fundamental part of the sexual tour.

There is also an erogenous zone **behind the knees** (many women apply perfume in this area). We must be particularly sensitive here: avoid nibbling, as this area is more sensitive to soft touches.

The **thighs,** the threshold to the genitals, constitutes a highly exciting area. Most of the blood deviates towards the capillaries, creating expectations for closeness and genital arousal. Massaging the thighs with a little oil or aromatic lotions will produce a very pleasant sensation.

Giving a relaxing **foot** massage will also provide pleasure. Move your fingers in circles, changing the direction of rotation from time to time. You can also use a piece of silk across the feet or utilize creams or oils.

And obviously the **genitals**: The **vagina** is also sensitive and houses the **G-spot** inside. This spot is named after the German gynecologist Ernest Grafenberg, who discovered it in 1960. The G-spot is a nubble about half a centimeter in diameter situated on the front of the vagina, between 2 to 4 inches inside. It is so sensitive because it is made of nerve endings, glands, and blood vessels. It only projects when touched directly, but it can sometimes be difficult to find. It can be stimulated by the penis during intercourse (the best position for this is when the man enters the woman from behind) or with your fingers. Interestingly, some women feel a sensation similar to needing to urinate when the G-spot is stimulated because this also puts pressure on the bladder.

The **perineum**, the area between the anus and the vagina, is usually an unexplored area but is also full of nerve endings, as it is formed by the same skin as the labia. It can be stimulated by stroking the area gently up and down or by pressing in circular movements.

The **anus** is also very sensitive even though the muscles that form it are much stronger than those of the vagina. This area may be uncomfortable for some women, but in this case, as in all cases, it is of utmost importance to use proper communication. The buttocks can also be stimulated with kisses, stroking, friction, etc.

The **vulva**, formed by the labia majora and minora, is extremely rich in nerve endings.

The **clitoris** is the most sensual, sensitive area for women (most women reach orgasm through stimulation). It must be done slowly (with fingers, mouth, tongue, etc.), stroking up and down or in a circular motion with a rhythm that the woman desires.

# The female deities

Tantric power is based on a trinity of competing and complementary forces: Shiva, Brahma, and Vishnu (masculine principles) have their mirrors in Kali, Laksmi, and Saraswat (female principles).

## Kali

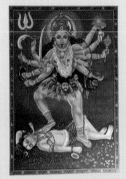

Kali represents the destruction and death of the ego. Kali's top right hand leads the sword that cuts off hypocrisy and the head of the ego; the top left hand holds the head that has been cut. The bottom right hand protects her devotees and eliminates fear. The lower left hand fulfills wishes and also represents the four cardinal points.

Kali is black, wild, and sticks out her tongue to show her sexual power, awake and unrestrained; her third eye is open and clearly visible. Her three eyes symbolize the past, present, and future. Kali is black, dark, and fully naked, as was the origin of the universe. Kali is and possesses kundalini energy and is completely active. Kali is the orgasmic wave in the female body.

Kali does not like selfishness, morality, envy, doubts, or fear, nor does she like hypocrisy, nor the masks of the ego. Of wild appearance, her inside is full of love and compassion.

Kali has the power of the sensual lover, extremely passionate. With a single look, she can ignite the skin, heart, and genitals of sensual men and women. Kali is the initiator of sexual mysteries. A woman who is identified with Kali has to know that she is a goddess of sexual action, without fear of taboos, and enjoys without conditions. She is open. Kali destroys everything that is unreal and grants wishes. Her pubis is black and bulky, natural and hairy.

When the woman eliminates contemporary false morals, obstacles and conditioning of the mind, she feels all of the splendor in your skin. Kali passion is stronger than prudish fear or the timidity of a submissive woman. The rites of Kali are performed during the dark cycle of the moon and during menstrual bleeding.

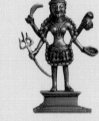

Kali revels in the sensual perfumes of sandalwood, musk, and patchouli. She likes red flowers, erotic dances, wine, and rhythmic drum music. These perfumes and elements enjoy being worshiped through every woman's body, as well as through their mantras, which are *Om namah Kali*, her proper name, the bija mantra (the syllable seed) *Hung*, and *Om namah kalika kang*.

## Lakshmi

The female counterpart of Vishnu, the Preserver, is the goddess Lakshmi. With a fresh and extremely fine look, Lakshmi is the stereotype of the loving,

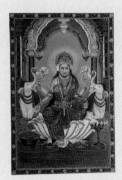

compassionate woman: tender, sensual, beautiful, and affectionate.

Lakshmi is the link to all that is the subtle and romantic, to love and emotion. Lakshmi governs the touch and contact between two sensual lovers.

Lakshmi expresses her affection, love, and desire. She stops time with her exquisite presence. Whenever you see a nice woman, you see Lakshmi right before your eyes. Whenever you receive a touch, a sweet smile, or a loving embrace, you will see Lakshmi through the exciting eyes of Shakti.

## Saraswati

She is the goddess of arts, culture, and dominion over the world. Saraswati, the eternal love of Brahma, is the figure of the intelligent, wise, and cultured woman. She can give advice and has experience with your life; she is adventurous and cautious. Saraswati is related to sound, hence why she is represented with a musical instrument.

Saraswati is the patroness of the 64 arts of Tantra. Through her music we can sample great charm. When a woman sings, dances, or performs an artistic work, it is the goddess Saraswati manifested.

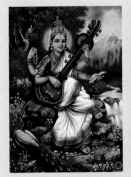

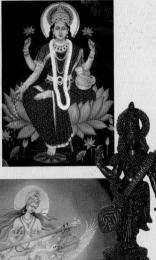

## Feminine freedom

The practice of Tantra gives you a release. Women question, "Of what should I free myself?" Firstly, of fears, chains, the mind, morality, guilt, conditioning, submission, and pain. Do not confuse this with debauchery; no one is claiming this lack of control, but an orderly freedom, consciously knowing what you want and what you need, which can often be different.

Submission, existential inertia, only serves to stop evolution, like to be a wilted flower or a blank, black box.

Sometimes, nourishment has a great deal to do with this state, in addition to character. It is certain that Shakti will undergo a revolution in your life when the kundalini energy, the treasure of life, is reserved and manifested in yourself. It is like the buds of the trees in spring or a bear coming out of hibernation or a sailboat that lifts its sails. Boost your wings, dance, enjoy, celebrate, breathe, mediate, and above all, empower your sexual life!

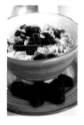

Sometimes, nourishment has a great deal to do with this state, in addition to character.

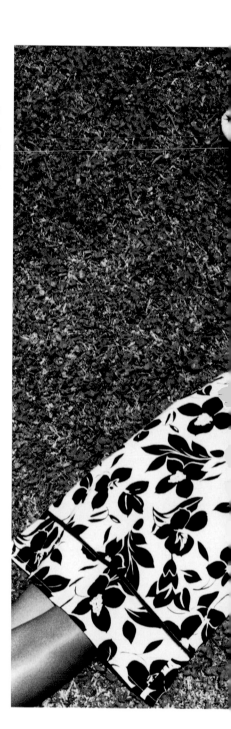

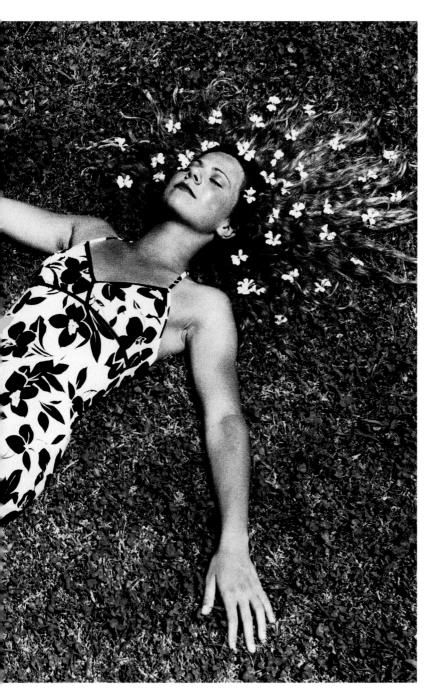

Shakti experiences a revolution through your life when the kundalini is reserved and manifested in yourself, like the buds of the trees in spring.

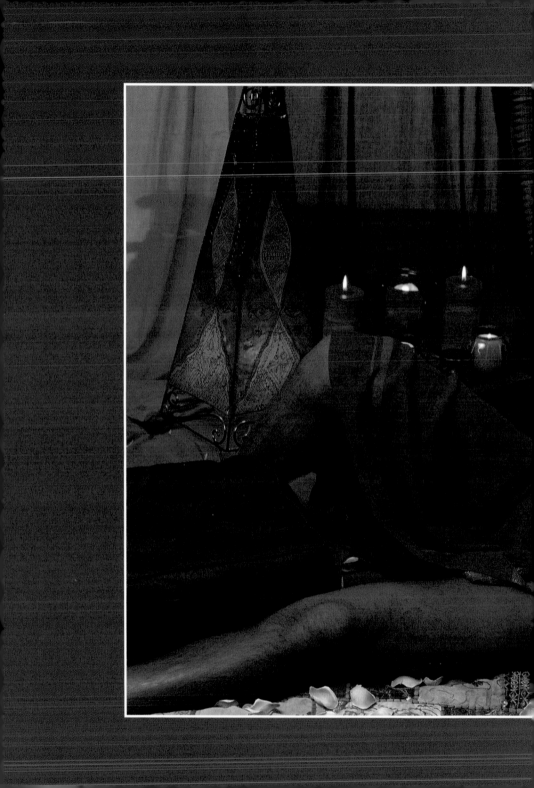

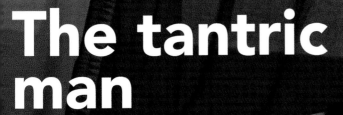

# The tantric man

*"Shiva is pure existence, the immortal divine principle. Shiva is pure, unconditional, and transcendent consciousness. Shiva is the diety of the mond, the lord of yoga, the teacher of the three worlds and conqueror of death. The entire universe was created by the Shakti of Shiva."*

SHIVA PURANA

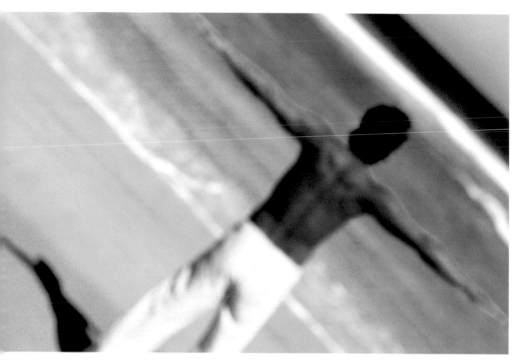

# Knowing the inner god

**Shiva is the creator of yoga, the supreme master of Tantra.**

*"Do not suppress your feelings; choose what you want and do as you wish, as this will please the goddess mode. Perfection can be achieved through the satisfaction of desire."*

GUHYASAMAJA TANTRA

Shiva is the cosmic Danzarin, the spinning motion of the planet life. Shiva is the creator of Yoga, the supreme master of Tantra. Shiva reveals the secrets of life to his Shakti. Shiva *knows*, due to pure experience; Shiva knows techniques and has been released.

Shiva has sensitivity and strength, combining magic and the caress, the art of sex and silence, the deployment of dance, and metaphysical wisdom.

And every man can (and should) awaken the attributes of Shiva. It is time to break away from the TV remote and take command of your personal existence. We cannot live on the earnings and victories of our favorite teams.

Women get fed up with men who waste an adventurous life in the routine of work, in watching hours of television, or in drinking with his friends. Find the maximum possible time to enjoy life with your lover and your life will experience a major change.

Women want fun, sexy, witty, sweet, and positive men. We cannot enslave ourselves to the category of "wife" (a cadence that suggests a removal of freedoms), as the woman who should always remain a mistress: **"lovers"** signifies "two who love each other"; **"spouses"** refers to being handcuffed (strung) together.

Throughout history, religions have been so pervasive in the lives of people, dictating rules of behavior that help to maintain social cohesion. This was done through a prism full of fears and almost facist moralizing.

In the case of Catholicism, the church forced people to generate a promise ("I will love you until the day you die") which now, for more than one reason, but mainly due to cultural and economic issues, is more difficult for anyone to meet. Actually, what should be said is, "I will love you until the day that love dies and the flower changes."

It may sound bad, but the reality is that most men are simply "human in the end." We are like bees in search of pollen: if you do not produce pollen, the bee will look elsewhere. For every man who has awakened the power of Shiva, the woman is a flower with an irresistible fragrance.

Personal relationships are an entire world, as pointed out in the Woody Allen film, *Annie Hall*:

"Doctor, my brother is crazy. He believes he is a chicken."

"Why don't you have him locked up?"

"I would, but I need the eggs."

Well, that's how I see relationships between people; completely absurd, but we maintain them because we need the eggs!

In Tantra, relationships are an art. Shiva is wise, pragmatic, subtle, and loving; every woman admires those qualities in a man: patient and sensitive at the same time. There is no need to demonstrate manhood with a strong handshake. You are a man and can demonstrate that with a tear. The silly stereotype of "men do not cry" has only managed to create a shield and armor.

The sun of Tantra warms the presence of Shiva in you; once you feel that you are a vibrating melody, a magnet that attracts, you create a love spell.

> Shiva is the cosmic Danzarin, the spinning motion of planets and life.

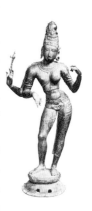

# Discover your multiorgasmic ability

In matters of sex and Tantra, there is an unprecedented idea being produced in the West. Magazines, books, and the media in general are addressing, with increasing sincerity, a subject that had been taboo: sex.

As far as I'm concerned, a while ago I wrote some articles for some widely disseminated men's magazines (*Men's Health, Playboy*, etc.) with the intention of spreading the art of Tantra. Now I am asked for many different collaborations. Why is that? I think it has to do with the current idea popular in the west, that a man can have an orgasm without ejaculating.

Men typically feel that if they do not ejaculate, something is missing. The Tantra always seek to remain "turned on." From the beginning, it says: "when the initial call comes, keep it, avoiding the embers towards the end."

This means we must always maintain being **on**: in a plane flying high in desire. And as we know, the ejaculation of desire weakens the lingam and organs. The senses are stunned, the dream appears, and magnetism disappears; the chance to return to the source "back home,"

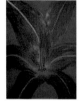

Prolong the fragrant sensitivity and maintains desire.

to the energetic drive, is lost. There was, yes, a physical response, a discharge of tension mixed with some pleasure. But the tantric know that an orgasm is another thing altogether. In order to understand: imagine for a moment what a room looks like with a sixty-watt bulb, intermittent dim light, illuminating very little. Now imagine a football stadium at night with all of their lights

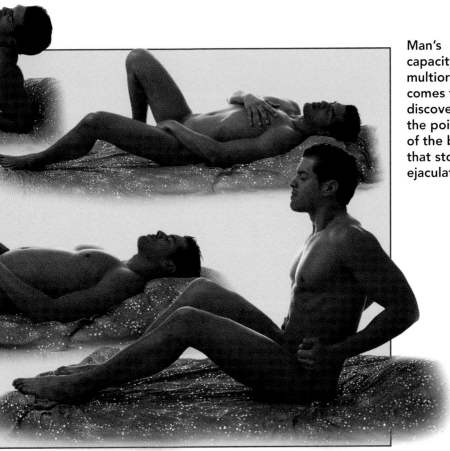

**Man's capacity for multiorgasms comes from discovering the points of the body that stop ejaculation.**

and ten thousand spectators chanting your name. The feeling is different, right? A brief burst of light in comparison with the continuous light from an orgasmic sun.

The man discovers his multiorgasmic capabilities by **defeating instinct with consciousness, knowing the points of the body** that stop ejaculation, using tantric **breathing** techniques to bring more air into the sexual fire, dominating **the mind** (which is the main sexual organ), and distributing electrical energy of sex throughout the body more globally and less centered in the genitals.

Forget being a stallion; you really don't have to leave the mark of semen on any woman creating a false illusion of possession; instead, plant tender and prolonged fragrances and keep your desire turned on throughout the day.

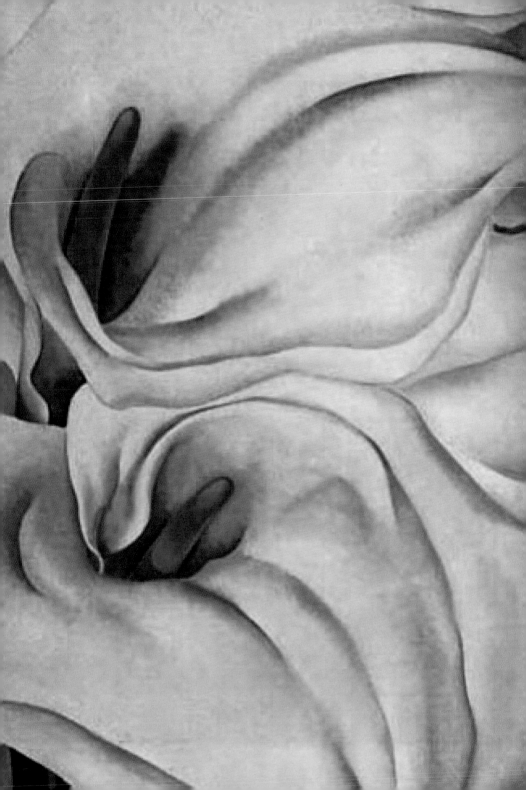

# Erotic points of the male body

As I mentioned, the man has to decentralize power from the genital area. The lingam has to be an engine to distribute the vibration from every pore and corner of the body. It is a **magic wand**, but you have to know how to use it; I do not mean moving it alternatively within a yoni, but to share his power with the spiritual pole on top of the head, the *Sahasrara* chakra.

From the lingam, the pole of animal-humankind, journeys toward the pole of divinity as the height of the fontanelle begins.

When you start to wake up, from the the the lingam (polarity yang), your navel (in contact with the feminine one), your breasts (the yin polarity), your mouth (sensual center), your hands (unfolding magnetism), your anus (male G-spot), and your testicles (bags of life), you'll know that your body is a sexual energy like an ocean current.

These points are loaded with enormous sexual electromagnetism when touched, kissed, sucked, or blown. You should stimulate them when you perform the *Meditation of the androgynous* with touching that excites your entire body while breathing and visualizing the serpentine flame. This will prepare you for *maithuna*. It is important that Shiva discovers these points alone, that he seeks mastery in the art of love and sex. Then, when your Shakti is present, light will have to be shared; you will know yourself because of your energy; you will empathize with female joy and will dissolve in a sea of sensations.

**Breathing** is essential to mastering the steed of sexual energy. Learning to breathe, you learn to slow down; stop and channel ejaculation and increase your personal power.

Many sexologists, ignorant of the wisdom of Tantra, say that not ejaculating is dangerous. Without a doubt, they know nothing of **energy channels** where the energy of

**These points are heavily loaded with sexual electromagnetism when touched.**

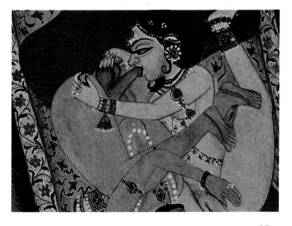

semen is transformed into spiritual energy (Shakti eyes), allowing not only the proper functioning of your prostate, but also your entire body.

More than 5,000 years of tantric wisdom consist of unmatched research dedicated to the hundreds of "scientific studies" that have proven to often be simple statistics of human deprivation because of a narrow and perverse vision of the scientific method (for some things, but is useful and powerful for others). It is the materialistic conception of Masters and Johnson, or of the Shere Hite reports.

In previous decades (Sigmund Freud, Wilhelm Reich), there was a logical reaction to knowing and deciphering a topic as important as this. We can say that, in general, these theories became valid to treat sexual issues with many traditional tools. However, in regard to the metaphysical, spiritual, and existential part of sexual energy, they could not contribute anything. Tantra is an invitation to experience; take the test and feel for yourself; it is the only reality that will you know because you have to experience in order to know.

Stimulate your erotic points, channel your energy, fill your skin with fire and your heart with peace, so sex will be your friend, not your master.

> Tantra is an invitation to experience; take the test and feel for yourself; it is the only reality that will you know because you have to experience in order to know.

## Increase your magnetism

Magnetism appears first through pheromones, your natural smell. Just as deers secrete a musk to stimulate females, your own scent can be your best ally. Please remember that you do not have to smell bad. Even today I cannot understand the fact that

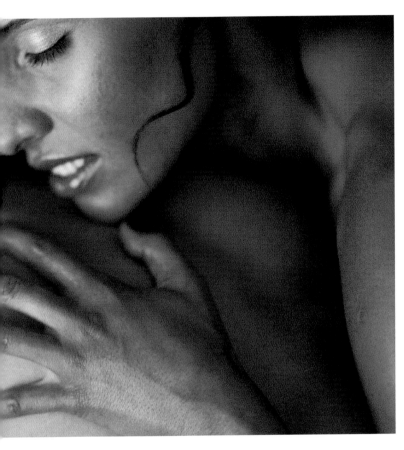

Stimulate your erotic points, channel your energy, fill your skin with fire and your heart with peace, so sex will be your friend, not your master.

there are many who disregard personal hygiene.

Tantra is an ally of the senses in all of its aspects; to increase your eroticism you can spread aphrodisiac oils all over your skin and thus enhance the power of your own natural scent. This method will only take you halfway, but you'll think that it really magnetizes the energy you emit, your personal vibration. From the quality of the food you eat to the way you chew and digest, through tantr' practices of energy elevation, you can have a constant gift of magnetic energy that will positively influence your quality of life, from business to sexuality.

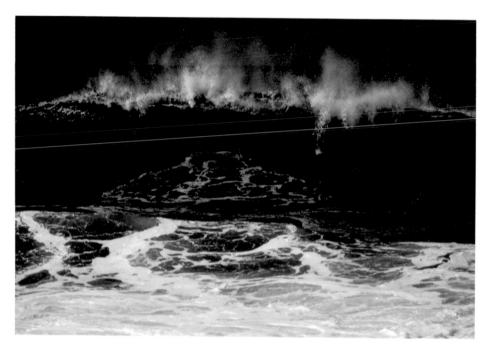

## The wisdom of sexual rhythms

**The wheel turns endlessly because you learn to reach the summit and travel down into the valley, up and down, holding an increasingly large winding fire.**

Man's energy is explosive, dynamic, and instant. This is because he has exterior genitals. Women, however, are introverted with genitals inside; they are deeply excited more slowly, but able to last longer.

The tantric man learns to also have a female pace, delivery, responsiveness, and openness. The known phases of excitement, plateau, orgasm, and resolution do not function as means of communication in Tantra.

The tantric sexual proposal is **seduction** (from the Latin *seducire*: "bringing the outside inside"),

light the fire, breathe consciously, awaken the senses, touch all the erogenous parts in order to strengthen them . . . And it is also enabled in chakras, connected with skin, games, penetration, free joy, orgasms, meditation, silence, immobility, changing positions to circulate energy through the body, opening consciousness, fullness, excitement, relaxation . . . there is a difference, right?

The wheel turns endlessly because you learn to reach the summit and travel down into the valley, up and down, holding an increasingly large winding fire. That journey can take hours! You can see, therefore, that this is very different than the few minutes you normally engage in sex.

One has to feel that the coitus is turned on all day! The face and hands will transmit their light that has kindled Kundalini energy.

Sometimes someone says, "But I've been unknowingly tantric." Clarify to them that to endure for hours without ejacluation is not tantric. Tantrism is a celebratory and holistic way of living life and is not limited to being an *exceptional* lover.

The tantric attitude is inclusive, positive, and does not divide, and goes well beyond the sexual episode. If we dig a little into expressions like "One thing is business and the other is spiritual" there is division. We must live spiritually in all acts, from money management to meditation.

The usual way a man finishes kills the pace and kills desire instantly. Therefore, if we have even a modicum of intelligence, we can see that we do not want that. Believe me, there is much more than what is known . . . .

**You have to live spiritually in all acts, from money management to meditation.**

---

# Three types of lingam

As the Bee Gees said in their album *Size Isn't Everything*, we should not be obsessed with penis size . . . . The *Kama Sutra* and the *Anaga Ranga* classify the lingam as having three functions.

**The Hare**
In this lingam, the erection is about 13 cm and is considered of a small dimension. Usually men with this lingam are short and quiet in character. His semen is sweet.

**The Bull**
This lingam measures around 22 cm and is considered medium-sized. These men are tall and hard-faced and enjoy making love at all times.

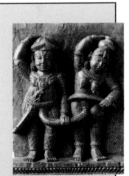

**The Horse**
This lingam is about 25 cm at full erection and is considered large. The man with this lingam is tall, muscular, and has a tendency towards food, passion, and sometimes laziness. Surprisingly, they have a calmer sexual desire. Their semen is rich and savory.

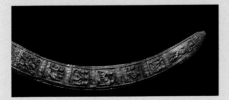

## Controlling ejaculation

In Tantra, it is important not to ejaculate because semen is considered to be a precious substance: Tantra teaches man not to ejaculate (or to do so less often) in order to preserve and better distribute his energy.

Although the widespread belief says otherwise, **man is able to control his own ejaculation;** this includes cases of "premature ejaculation" (specialists disagree on the criteria for this: for some, it is premature ejaculation if done so before initiating intercourse, while for others it refers to ejaculating before his partner does so).

Regardless of these differences, it is important to control ejaculation. To do this, man must learn to know his body and its feelings, which traditionally does not happen. **It is about learning to read signals that our body gives while we are on our way to orgasm** (especially when approaching the end), to know and to interpret them without losing eroticism or excitement.

That is the basic premise of **the first technique**, known as **the pause**. This consists of stimulating your penis (you can have a woman do this, but we should first have the man do so himself) as if masturbating, reaching the maximum degree of excitement. In that moment, the man should stop and wait to decrease the sense before ejaculating (there is no concrete time for this; for some it may be half a minute, while for others, it may be a minute and a half). It is normal for the erection to go down slightly, even 50%. Then the man should continue the same stimulation before stopping at the same time as previously. He should repeat this three times; during the fourth time, he can go all the way to ejaculation. This is perfectly normal. Sometimes a man will ejaculate earlier than expected. The important part is that he learns to know which sensations precede orgasm and how to control them.

Controlling ejaculation is similar to controlling urination. Hence, if we learn to control the feeling of urination, we can advance. You have to train the pubic muscles, contracting

### Unsuitable methods

Some think that **to delay ejaculation** (although delaying is not the same as controlling) one should imagine some less erotic scenes—think about work, recite the alphabet or a team's roster, or even bite your own lip. All this does is keep you from experiencing pleasure. It is counterproductive to think of other things because this means decreasing control over the signals that announce ejaculation. Ointments, anesthetics, creams, or other products sold by catalogs or "sex shops" are really effective.

and relaxing them. The simplest way is to learn which muscles allow us to stop urinating. Once learned (a slight contraction of the anal sphincter and pelvic muscles), you can train anywhere.

**Breathing is also very important in controlling ejaculation**. If we learn to breathe deeply, we can learn to also distribute energy throughout the body and not just the genitals. It should be like the breathing of a locomotive: quickly inhaling and exhaling through the mouth, panting like an animal.

Tantra also teaches **several pressure points in our bodies** that can help control ejaculation. For example, **the man can press two fingers against a point two inches above his nipple while exhaling completely**. You can also **press the perineum** (the point between the anus and the testicles), although this method is perhaps too mechanic.

One of the teachings of Tantra to control ejaculation is to

**bring the tongue up to the palate**: bend the tongue back to close the threshold of orgasm.

**Another way to control ejaculation is known as "the grip."** It is similar to the pause, but in this case you press your thumb and index finger against where the heart begins right at the moment when the man begins to feel that ejaculation is inevitable. This, again, is a mechanical method and can lose the mood of the moment.

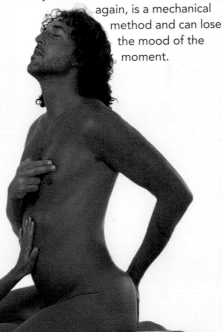

## Male deities

As I said, the three goddesses have their male counterparts:

### Shiva

Shiva is the dancer of the cosmos. He embodies the aspect of destruction, destroying in order to create something new and improved. It is the law of evolution. The energy of Shiva destroys armor in order to create a new being, destroys an old house to build a new one with the energy of Brahma.

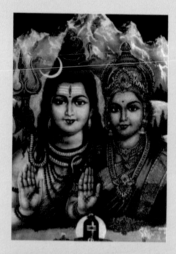

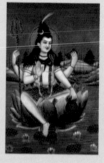

When something is destroyed in our lives, latent energy is created. Shiva is the mobility and every man who invokes this energy uses it for personal evolution; you are able to advance step by step by making interior changes. "If you do not become like a child, you cannot enter the Kingdom of Heaven," as Jesus said. Unless you destroy your emotional armor and obstacles of your personality, you will not see the essence of your pure and eternal being.

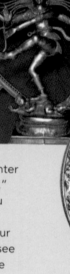

In the physical body of Shiva is the vital energy and breath; in the subtle body, the Sushumna channel, the center is where the divine kundalini shakti meets Shiva, at the top of the head. Shiva is also called "The Transcendental."

## Brahma

The divine creation. He is the energy of the creative process, of making things, the aspect of creative energy. All men who identify and invoke the energy of Brahma will flow with a creative vibration that permeates all of life. It is an illusion to think that the creator made the world in only seven days. Creation for Tantra is a constant process: new flowers and fruits, new children, new buildings, everything is moving and changing, everything is recreated again and again, evolving. His strength allows the birth of all beings.

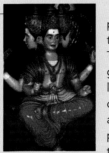

Brahma is the subtle body of pingala nadi, corresponding to the right nostril, hot and male. The symbol of Brahma is a golden egg, an aura of magnetic light. Brahma governs the destiny and the world. Brahma also represents food in the physical body. To be Brahma is to really be creation and flow in harmony. In the ancient times of Abraham (a: negative particle; brahma: the creator), maybe the tribe that went with Abraham was the one that moved away from Brahma.

## Vishnu

Brahma creates, Shiva destroys, and Vishnu preserves creation. His divine role is conservation. Vishnu is the keeper who maintains works. In the energetic body, Vishnu conserves the proper functioning of the Ida canal, the lunar duct, that has its counterpart in the left nostril. He is the matriarchal force and is also known as the Lord of Water because water governs all. The symbol of Vishnu is a seashell and is associated with eroticism (as saliva, relating to the erotic and water element). In governing the water,

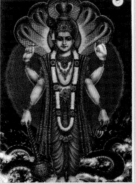

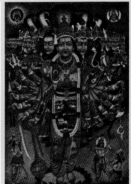

this god generates, together with Lakshmi, the preservation of life. In agreement with ancestral Hindu myths, Kama (the god of love and desire) is the son of Vishnu and Lakshmi.

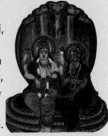

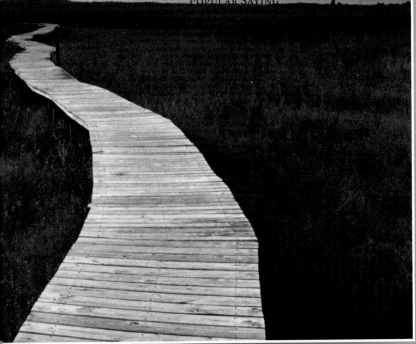

# Tantra, the beautiful way

*"Beauty is in the eye of the beholder."*

<small>POPULAR SAYING</small>

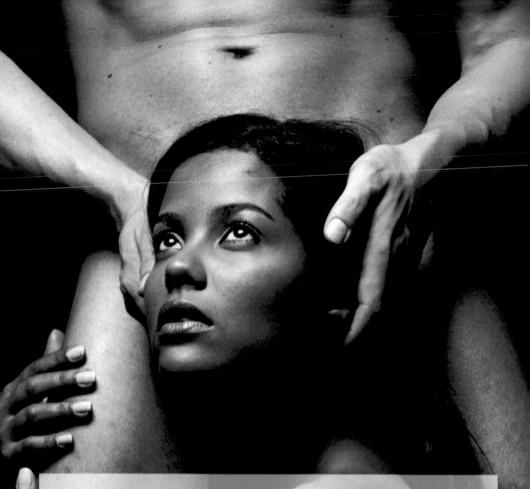

# The wonder of the body

The body is the container for the soul and the laboratory where we transform energy and consciousness. It is also the place where we can plant seeds of pleasure or thorns of pain, of martyrdom, and of bad habits. Everyone knows that there are "cultural" events, which really are aberrations, such as clitoridectomy or self-flagellation with whips. Tantra is the path of pleasure and beauty: accept the body and care for it, worship it, love it. We do not care if the vehicle cannot take us far. All of the functions of the body are perfect, as it was designed in a state of homeostasis to occur permanently. However, for strange reasons, there are also bad habits tha the body can overcome like being ill or weakened. We need to think about our roles, to bring energy to our organs, mucles, and bones. Tantra inscribes a poem on the body as it is the first stage of our spirital development. This story contains our personal history from birth and carries the stigma attached to our lives including our emotions, actions, and habits.

Besides, anyone who practices physical exercise or yoga knows how the body is after activity. When energy moves throughout the meridian network, it feeds on blood and energy and all systems are revitalized.

Take care of the body with essential oils through automassage or massaging between two or more tantric practitioners: immerse in baths with salts and minerals, take dynamic showers, sleep, be full of energy and activity, rub essential oils into the skin, have sex, meditate, do yoga, dance, bathe in the sun, practice technical breathing, enjoy jacuzzis and saunas, and keep a positive attitude and posture at work . . . everything contributes to establish a program of care that will nourish the body from all possible angles. Do not ignore signals from the body or its desires and needs. There is a similar manner of speaking that talks about pain that occurs when this energy flow is blocked.

Tantra is not oriented to narcissism or comparing abs at the beach; it is more interested in the physical fitness involved with overall health. Everything else is pure consequence and is not the end we seek.

The body is art, poetry in action, but is also a mystery. The origin of man goes back millenniums and we do not know if we came from mud, aliens, or what actually happened. Have you ever wondered who cared for the first baby? Did Adam just appear as an adult of 30? Who nursed him? Who cared for him? Didn't he need supervision? It is a mystery . . . .

But as Osho says, "The mysteries are to be lived, not solved." He adds, "The body is a great mechanical device, the greatest. It has millions and millions of cells and each is alive. So you are a city of sixty trillion cells; there are approximately sixty trillion citizens within you and the whole city works very quietly without problems. This mechanism is operating at every moment."

In Tantra, we live with pure pleasure in this life because our origin is pleasure and we return to a great pleasure when we complete our destinies. Meanwhile, at the time we are alive, we decide to nurture our intelligence and learn from our body, which is certainly a great teacher.

**The body is art, poetry in action, but is also a mystery.**

**We come into the world naked, innocent, wise, open, and receptive.**

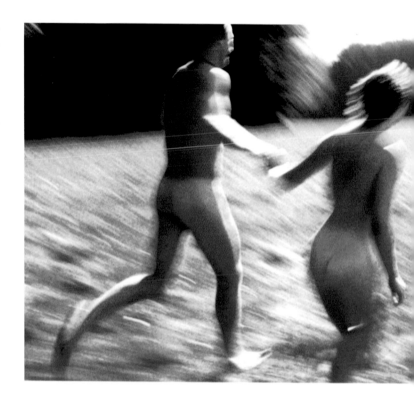

## Naturalness

For Tantra, nudity is something natural, without mental connotations; there is no shame or hinderance. We come into this world nude, innocent, wise, open, and receptive. The body and soul are a level table until they start to embrace all kinds of conditions. Why do Muslims hide the divine and beautiful face of women? The face, like the female body, is a delight, a treat for the eyes—why conceal it? Why fear the sensual look of a woman? It is simple: a woman can make a man lose his head with only a look. By only transmitting fire, eroticism, and sensuality through the eyes or a gesture, men might lose all control, become aroused, get an erection, or become crazy about her: is this not the story of humanity? From Cleopatra to Helen of Troy, from Joan of Arc to Lady Di, from Madonna to Sophia Loren, women have generated revolutions with their seduction, their power, and their beauty; thus many

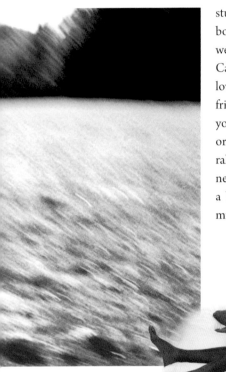

students are grateful. Touching a body is touching the divine, since we are a replica of the supreme. Caress your naked body and your lover; venerate them. Start to be friends with your nakedness and you will gradually return to your original state of freedom and naturalness. Tantra means that the connection between body and spirit is a bridge that cannot disappear, as much as we would like it to; only

**In the courses of Tantra, we feel that nudity breaks unnatural walls and students are grateful.**

men prefer to censor their divinity, which is a clear sign of inferiority.

Tantra removes all veils and deceit and accepts how natural we are. Obviously, we dress to shelter ourselves, but at home, why can we not enjoy the naked body? Those who go to nude beaches know the unmatched feeling of being naked in the water or under the sun; this produces a tremendous psycho-emotional release. In the courses of Tantra, we feel that nudity breaks unnatural walls and

in the last exhalation does the soul travel to another world and body and concludes its mission; therefore it has quit naturally from your life.

*Author's Note: I would like to comment on something magical for readers who understand how the fabric of Tantra works. When I finished writing this section about the benefits of the naked body, my phone rang and I was asked to teach Tantra in the nudist village in Catalonia. Remember, the universe is alive and listens to the heart.

## Bodies and faces in ecstasy

Our origin is ecstasy, the explosion of a cosmic orgasm. We are children of the great universal pleasure of creation, at a macrocosmic level, and the small pleasure of our parents, at a microcosmic level. We can live in constant ecstasy if we understand that the Earth and this life are gifts, but we lose these gifts because of either concerns of the future or attachments of the past. John Lennon fantastically recorded, "Life is what happens while you are busy making other plans."

**If your body is in ecstasy, with closed eyes you can enter paradise within.**

After practicing Tantra, faces reflect the peace and fullness within. Tantra does not create tension, but creates and excites

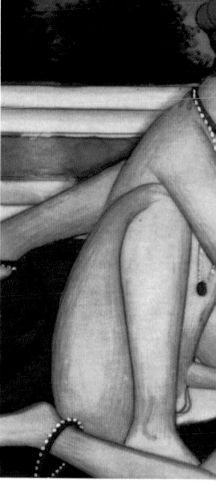

sexual energy while managing it with deep, natural channels; so it flows from the nervous system to the chakras, from the muscles to the soul. Outward expressions like fire in the eyes are manifestations of the fire in the heart. If our souls are full

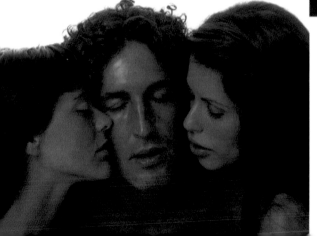

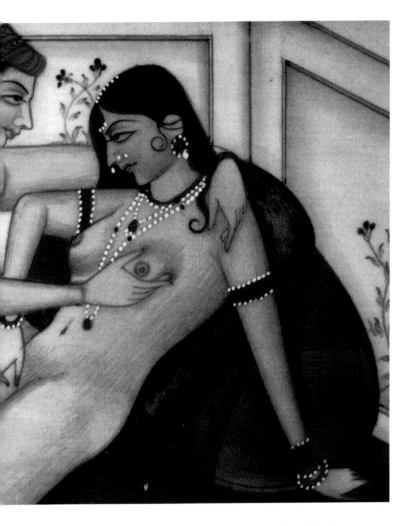

External expressions such as fire in the eyes will be manifested from fire in the heart.

of excitement, connection, pleasure, and fullness, and our desires are satiated through transmitting spiritual and emotional sexual energy, our faces will reflect it.

If you look into the eyes of others, you will know what is inside. Carefully see their physical expressions and you will be able to read their body. A body in ecstasy and peace is loaded with energy; some do not need gesturing to prove it. It is correct that a simple gesture can provoke an emotion; a hand, awaken sensitivity; a look, unleash the greatest excitement. With eyes closed, you can be led into your inner paradise.

**We will have a trip with life; we will swim in the current, flow, and fly every day.**

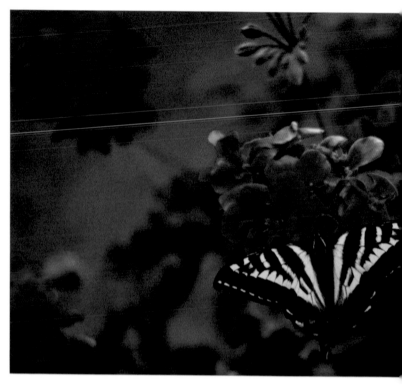

## Understanding reality

There is a Reality with capital letters and another with lowercase letters: your reality. Reality is the eternal present and is available at all times; life flows. Your reality has beliefs, habits, taboos, tricks, addictions, desires, concerns, emotions, masks, breastplates, ego . . . .

The highest Reality is naked, devoid of boundaries. In order to distinguish this Reality from our personal reality we have to mute

the mind through meditation and through observation of our lives. Most problems are imaginary, they can happen, the keys are in your imagination . . . but they do not really exist. For example, do you fear someone breaking in and robbing your house (even if it's never happened)? Scared that a lover might leave you, although it's not possible? Are you afraid that your parents will die, but they are alive and kicking? There are thousands of examples. The reality is that we are well, that we have the opportunity to change our destinies

enter the meditative and ecstatic state that provides practice, while leaving that which emits fear or morality in the periphery of the mind, and don't feel anything. It's not that Tantra does not have an effect, but we will be tied to our chains unless we are willing to fly. Tantra gives us wings, but if we do not jump, nothing will happen. Tantra is not a cure-all or a pill that allows us to do miraculous things. Tantra gives you the vehicle, a Formula One race car that can reach 350 mph, but you have to drive!

**Tantra gives wings, but if you do not jump, nothing will happen.**

through choice and that we can do so wisely with our discernment, but the problem is that there is fear. Fear paralyzes and is the opposite of the active power of love. We need to understand that our reality is actually fabricated by ourselves and if we reconcile with the higher Reality, the journey will make us one with life; we will swim in the current, flow, and fly every day. Tantra teaches us this.

My experience in the seminars has taught me that the people without these constraints readily

## Hindrances to practicing Tantra

Here is a brief list of hindrances to practicing Tantra. It is best to enter with humility and without expectations—loose and "mindless"—for this is the tantric light that can project to all corners of your being.

1. The mind, with its beliefs, habits, and pseudo-moralism
2. Fear
3. Religious constraints
4. Shyness and shame
5. Disease
6. Excuses
7. A possessive partner
8. Poor body image
9. Rushing
10. Expectations

> Religion is the symbol of misused power, a great business of selling land in an illusory, future heaven.

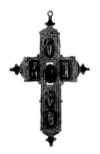

## Tantra and religion

The word "religion" comes from "re-linking" (back together), but Tantra understands that it is not possible to unite what cannot be separated. It is an illusion to think that we can be separated from the divine. The tantric vision is that everything is linked together in a cosmic matrix that has no limits. You cannot go outside because, in fact, there is no outside; everything is inside. In the first film of the *Matrix* trilogy, there is a small glimpse of that idea.

So if it is not a religion, what is it? Tantra is a spiritual path that unites mystical practices, sex, and the meditative light formed from a scientific way, towards personal development. This is different than dogmas and constraints, commandments and mortifications, in order to obtain a future paradise. The biggest difference is that religion makes every effort to make sure that *after* death, one enters a supposed paradise. Tantra's emphasis is on changing mortification through delight and future paradise through the present divine, because the Lord God is listening and available now.

Most of the wars arise because of different religious beliefs. Have you ever given any thought to barbarism? When you go to the mosque, synagogue, or church, remember those same people lynched everyone who didn't agree with their ideas...religion is the symbol of misused power, a great business of selling land in an illusory, future heaven.

## Repairing a broken heart, good-bye blame!

Betraying a heart, with feelings, emotions, love, and affection is going against life because life is a big heart, an open flower, a golden sunrise that is recycled.

Many people who have loved have suffered and do not want to return for fear that it will happen again. Without doubt, the human heart that has been injured can be repaired in the same way as the character Pinocchio. In the first place, he had to accept that he was not broken, but hurt and that wounds will heal. Healing provides new energy to those areas that are lacking. Tantra has a beautiful teaching: "With the same leg with which you fall, also lifts you up." This means that if the heart is broken, your mood is low; you have to uplift

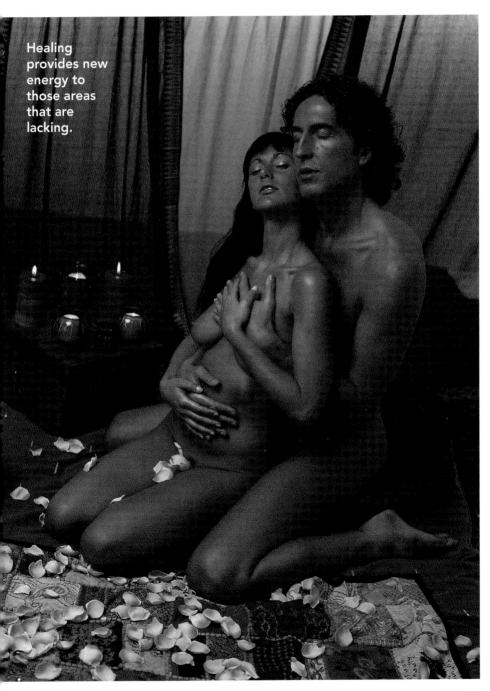

Healing
provides new
energy to
those areas
that are
lacking.

it to the heart. It is of alchemy, of transformation, but it does not happen magically; you have to act, perform, and modify your approach. Suffering is a great teacher, but hold it in your fist during instruction, and then one day open your hand and it will fly away like a bird. Often guilt prevents the heart from healing; you must drop everything that remains of your suffering so you can navigate the waters and shift towards a new horizon.

A simple but profound exercise I learned from Alejandro Jodorowsky, the creator of psychomagic, is to take a bag and fill it with stones. Each stone symbolizes something you want to remove from your life: jealousy, envy, resentment, a bad relationship, etc. According to the "weight" of these emotions, you choose a heavier or lighter stone and then fill the bag with as many stones as it takes.

Then you bring the bag along with you for a day. Go to the bathroom, to work, shopping . . . become aware of the load that you carry. You will sweat, curse, and feel uncomfortable, but do not let it go at any time.

**Suffering is a great teacher, but hold it in your fist during instruction, and then one day open your hand and it will fly away like a bird.**

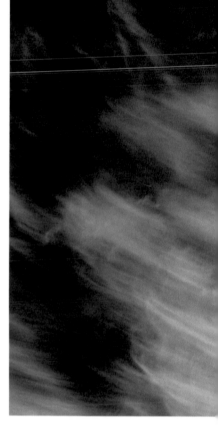

## Too much heaven

There are lots of paradises, many heavens, available, but right now, day to day, choose where you want to live. Heaven is an inner state, an infinite opening of joy and light. Your personal heaven

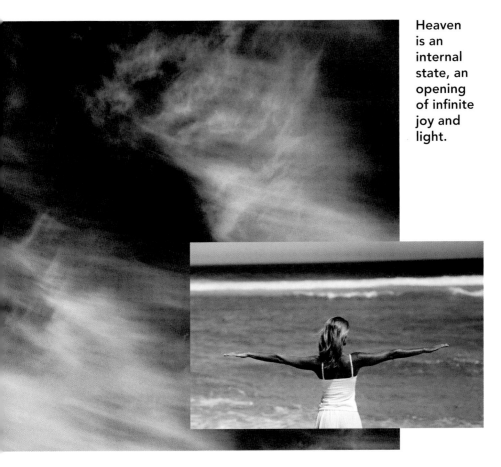

**Heaven is an internal state, an opening of infinite joy and light.**

can grow larger based on your own conscience; it's within you like an bomb of ecstasy that might explode at any time, and when that happens...there is light! That is why there are so many people on spiritual paths: they miss their homes, the place where consciousness expands and they become one. They find that they have the entire universe within themselves. There are many mental clouds that come down, many storms to cross until the clear sky is revealed in their beings.

Many times we don't know it, in the same way as a bow is drawn more and more until you shoot the arrow and loosen the string; when you release suffering you will achieve this same objective; you arrive at your inner center.

# A superior civilization

On a trip to Mexico, I soaked up the exciting culture of the Mayans. According to their sound mathematical investigations, mystics, astronomy, and geography, their codices says that in the year 2012 (on exactly December 12th), there will start a new era of light that will end the dark cycle and start a new, superior civilization. This coincides with the Easter (tantric) view, the era of Kali.

This planetary change will also bring important adjustments into the consciousness of humanity.

Therefore, it is desirable to properly prepare now through meditative practices and the proper use of sexual energy. There are some points about the Mayan culture that have been misinterpreted, such as the ballgame and the sacrifices. What does this have to do with tantric sex? First we must remember that for Tantra, life is a game, played with balls the size of planets revolving around the sun. The tantrics and Mayans called this game "Lilah," and it represented a spiri-

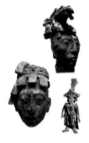

The Mayans speak of December 12th, 2012 as a great change in collective awareness.

**The goddess Kali holds a head in her hand to symbolize the death of the personal ego.**

tual and sexual initiation in their ball game. Candidates came from far away to learn these supreme mysteries. But it appears that those who were lost were sacrificed. Wait. The word "sacrifice" comes from *sacro* (sacred) and "craft" (work)—that is, they had a sacred job, but what was it? Well, it was using sexual energy. It is normally believed that being lost is like being beheaded, right? Well, politics and religion have hidden the truth through the following: How do you evangelize to highly evolved beings and connect them with the divine at all times? How do you talk about something they already know and talk about often? You gently let them be as uneducated barbarians; tell them they are wild and promiscuous. The Mayans performed sexual rituals; temples and phallic architecture prove this, but they collapsed. Likewise, the goddess Kali holds a head in her hand symbolizing the death of the personal ego. Mayans also symbolically cut the head (with all of the unnatural thoughts the head has provided) in order to

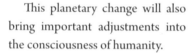

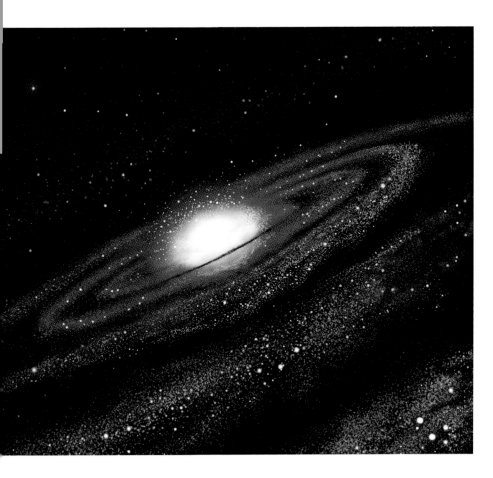

enter the greatest mysteries from the heart and mind. The reality is that the guillotine or hanging had no symbolic-esoteric meaning . . . .

The Mayans had techniques to awaken the third eye from a very young age: they placed a stone of gopal (intensive perfumed incense) on the forehead. Thus, the ajna chakra woke from childhood, activating the inner wisdom and clear vision. I do not intend to overthink this sacred culture, but only to comment that throughout history there have been many different manipulations to maintain this civilization "under control," but times change and repression falls. Do you prepare for a better civilization?

**For Tantra, life is a game, played with balls the size of planets revolving around the sun.**

## Living eyes, extrasensory perception. Do you think like your lover?

You will be surprised to know that the channelling of sexual energy increases many inner faculties in you and your lover. This is because it is generating a fuel called "Shakti Eyes," a kind of vital oil that begins to circulate throughout the body.

By not taking out the huge and powerful sexual energy through ejaculation, this triggers a magnetism that feeds the internal power (siddhis). For example, it is customary to practice tantric sex to awaken telepathy since energy is channeled. Thus, it is common to sense what the other thinks; think of someone and at that moment they call you on the telephone; or sense (see inside) that something will happen.

**By not taking out the huge and powerful sexual energy through ejaculation, this triggers a magnetism that feeds the internal power (siddhis).**

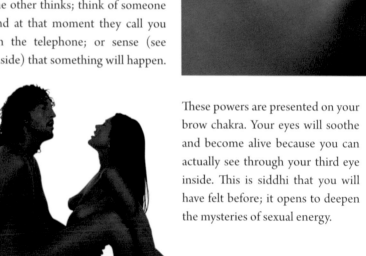

These powers are presented on your brow chakra. Your eyes will soothe and become alive because you can actually see through your third eye inside. This is siddhi that you will have felt before; it opens to deepen the mysteries of sexual energy.

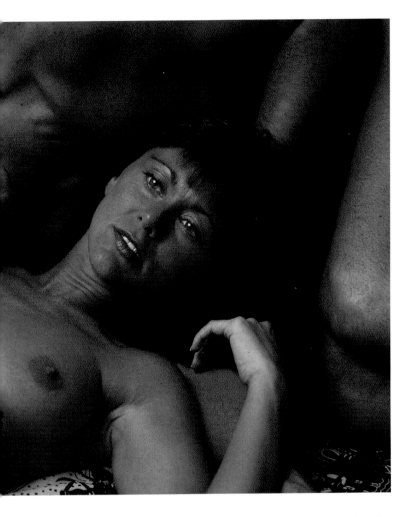

Your eyes will soothe and become alive because you can actually see through your third eye inside.

## One

We are one. We all respond to the same essence—the same life force that makes a heartbeat, the beating of all mankind. There is a cosmic heartbeat, and "cosmos" mean "order." There is an order behind all of this apparent chaos and it is nothing without the source, the

One before the Big Bang, before the duality. We are all interdependent cells of unity. The feeling of separation or duality arises from your ego. Take the test: do not do anything for an entire day, but only take notes. You will see that everything still works well, but if your activity is creative, positive, and joyous,

**The wind of consciousness will propel you forward and you'll find that you are navigating an eternal ocean of life and joy.**

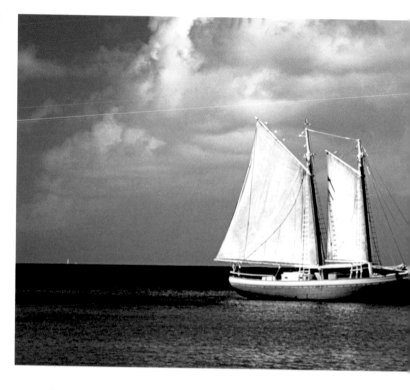

you will increase order! That is, that you only have part of the profits, because if you put a time bomb in the moment, things will return to the natural order, but if you make an invention, paint a picture, write a book, love someone, or enjoy your work, you will be collaborating. Thus, you are important and this unity opens doors.

Unity cannot be destroyed with chaos; in the same way that when you turn the switch on a light switch the darkness disappears instantly, unity can be increased.

Saint Exupery, the writer of *The Prince*, says, "Love is the only thing that increases when it is shared with others," and Hermann Hesse, author of *Siddhartha*, mentions, "Feel the unity everywhere, breathe; in this resides the supreme knowledge."

Tatric sex's main objective is to feel united, but not only physically united, but through sex, to feel the first unity, the genesis, two bodies with a single consciousness. Every man and woman has the intrinsic power (increased through practice) to enter the wisdom of unity.

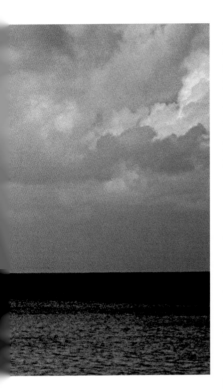

Artists become immortal by leaving a legacy to humanity. Art is a spiritual path that everyone has within himself. You can be creative in any activity that you do; there is a way to immortalize your passage through this life. But there is another, more profound way to enter eternity.

It is widely believed that if something is eternal, it was in the past, will be in the future, and therefore must also be in the present. And right now is when we have the opportunity to illuminate our souls in the light of eternity. If you feel that inside you are eternal, you'll never die and all fear disappears. The death of the body leaves to be a ghost and it takes on the form of a game in order to manifest itself. Each person has his or her own way, a personal history. Eternity is available and its doors open inside you with meditation, and much more with sexual meditation, because the energy of life is awake, it is a blossom of the soul, it is the boat with which you navigate in the eternal waters as their sails are deployed. The wind of consciousness will propel you forward and you'll find that you are navigating an eternal ocean of life and joy.

"Love is the only thing that increases when it is shared."

## Immortality

Skeptics say that when you die there is nothing left of you. You could argue that if there is nothing, there won't remain an "I" to feel anything . . . so why worry?

For Tantra, just as in many Eastern cultures, it is not as important where we come from or where we go, but who we are. Immortality is now available in the soul. The physical body will one day die, but the spirit will continue its journey through other planes.

# With tantric sex, you should be dancing

*Dance is produced in the heart; when you dance, you feel alive, enthusiastic, cheerful, full, at peace, and have a smile on your face.*

Many people complain of a lack of energy. There is only one energy, and it has many functions; when the body receives the energy produced from tantric sex, it creates such momentum, such contentment, and such fulfillment that all of the cells, chakras, and physical and psycho-emotional functions get to dance, to celebrate, to enjoy.

Life is a dance; remember Shiva, the lord of the yogis, the father Tantra, is the supreme dancer. When we dance, not only physically but emotionally, when we see everything as a harmonious symphony, our spirits become rigid, dry, and finally breaks through the swamps of bitterness.

I put a hand on your shoulder and tell you that you have a destination, that you have a gift; use it. Join the cosmic dance and feel that you are an important piece to increase the symphony.

In dance workshops, dancing occupies a key role and plenty of people do not know how you can end up dancing naked in front of others. It seems unnatural to remove layers down to our essence, but we feel that nudity is something totally natural. I am excited to

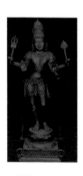

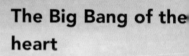

## The Big Bang of the heart

Our souls want to evolve, grow, and feel. The symbol of life, the supreme connection, days and nights, centuries and lives, can be found just around the corner. The journey begins and ends here. The heart hits a beat and life transforms.

Colors are not the same, smells and sounds, everything changes when the heart has an implosion to tap into the world, flowers, and music. Find the bridge to the cosmos to find your vision to the tenth floor, the moon, the sky full of stars, the wind on your naked body. Everything seems to make sense. The heart understands silence, the light is shared, and the magic and mystery of the supreme between the heart, breath, touch, movement, voices, and sighs.

see the progress of my students. I remember one of them told the group, "For a long time, I didn't do anything. I came from a difficult time, emotionally difficult. After I began practicing Tantra, one day I got up in the morning and looked

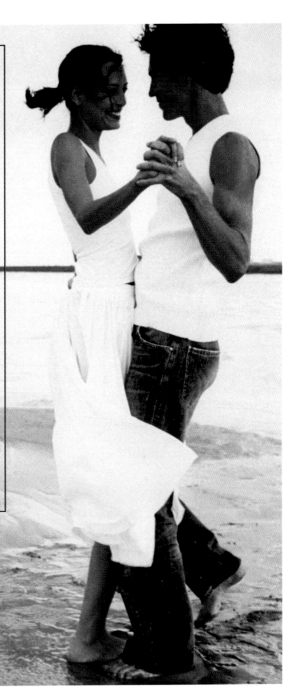

The serpentine fire accelerates, dances, and rises. The heavens are yours.

The soul celebrates only one, intertwined with each star. The drums beat, the blood boils passionately. Promises of the heart go to the depths of the night.

Reality of the soul, infinite relaxation, deep awareness.

God and goddess, two in one, instruments of love. Love makes you, transforms you, molds you; flow in a sea of sensations.

When the heart has its big bang, the orgasmic explosion of Life is in you.

in the mirror. For the first time in a long time, I felt a smile on my face." The dance is produced in the heart; when you dance, you feel alive, enthusiastic, cheerful, full, at peace, and have a smile on your face.

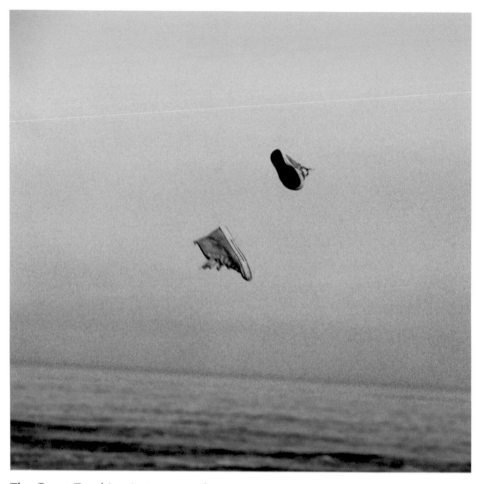

The Great Teaching is to surrender.
Surrender your control and let the whole
take you away wherever it would like to
take you . . . .

# Surrender

Osho says, "The Great Teaching is to surrender. Surrender your control and let the whole take you away whereever it would like to take you. Do not swim against the current. Let yourself be carried away by the river, become the river. The river is already going to the sea. This is the Great Teaching, the Mahamudra."

Einstein also said, "I think 99 times and I find nothing. I stop thinking and the answer appears." It is a paradox, right? We believe that if we don't do everything, it all falls apart as if nothing will happen without our effort. Obviously, if you have a business, you must devote a lot of energy to it, but in regards to teaching, surrendering is the appropriate attitude; be rendered to the ultimate, to focus away from the ego that thinks it is the center of the universe. In tantric sex, surrender is important—surrendering to our senses and to our desire to each other. Through surrender, the door is open and divinity can flow like the wind. If you stay in control, keeping tension, doing things your way, you'll lose the magic of surprise. If you have an attitude of surrender, it will be easier to give because in surrendering, to give is to share.

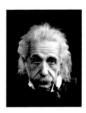

Einstein said, "I think 99 times and find nothing. I stop thinking and the answer appears."

## The Tantric Lover's Prayer

Love lights up my life like the morning lights the world. I let the ocean of life come to me and flow freely.

Happiness lives with me forever; I smile freely. Love is my energy, the spiritual sun that feds me. I have peace of mind.

I have a fire in my spirit. I'm alive and I celebrate and sing. I am a lamp that shines beyond punishment or failures.

I am strong like the sun, calm as a lake, and powerful as fire.

I am as peaceful as the breeze in the spring, but rebellious as a child.

Let the power of my soul manifest in every action. Everything my eyes see today will make me smile. If asked why, I'll say that I'm happy.

It sends messages of joy, radiates peace, salutes to the past and future, and breathes in the nectar of the eternal present.

I feel that I am immortal, traveling through eternity.

I transform my life into a party, I feel full, free, and I will make all of my wishes come true.

The Universe is on my side. I know that if I work for love, my time in the world will have a feeling. I lift this prayer to Creation and am grateful to live another day with awareness, enthusiasm, and creativity. This magic is my manifesto. I breathe happiness.

Surrender control of your mind with all of its conditioning towards your body, heart, and freedom.

To scale the heights of conscience and spiritual elevation, you need to let go of that which binds you and keeps your soul from growing. Just as a rocket detaches itself from some of its parts in order to reach the moon, so must the intrinsic human spirit detach itself.

## How deep is your love?

There are two basic ways to live: being in love or not being so. Love is the energy that fuels the engine and humanity. Life makes colors of love, with intense vibration, and bubbling with loving unity. On the path of love grows flowers, but also weeds. It is a workout, a constant give and take that expresses love, like a plant, requiring care and attention. We often confuse sex with love. There are many people that, until you spend more time with them or complete a routine of movies, dinners, walks, etc., will not make love, or rather, have sex with the "unknown." Each person is different; some may have sex within a few hours of knowing each other while others need more time. So the question arises: is there such a thing as love at first sight? Of course! If you are receptive you will be able to feel it; this is available any time. Life is the power of love.

Often attraction appears first, which is inescapable because it is a law of energy.

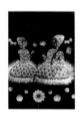

**It is training, a constant give and take because love, like a plant, requires care and attention.**

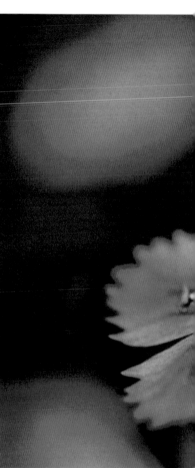

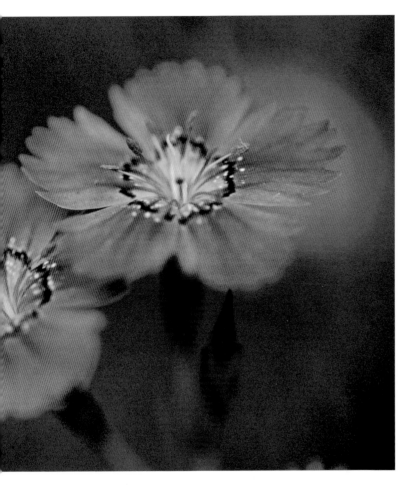

**You feel attracted to someone because you want to love and love overflows.**

Even after ten years of being married, you will still be able to attract other beings. There are only three ways to take human energy: indifference, repulsion, and attraction. There cannot only be attraction without love, but also attraction with love. Love is the impulse to love the other, cuddle, kiss, caress, protect, laugh, release, experience . . . . You feel attracted to someone because you want to love and love overflows, because you can feel it from any direction. The problem is when your heart is blocked or closed; you cannot love until you clear it out.

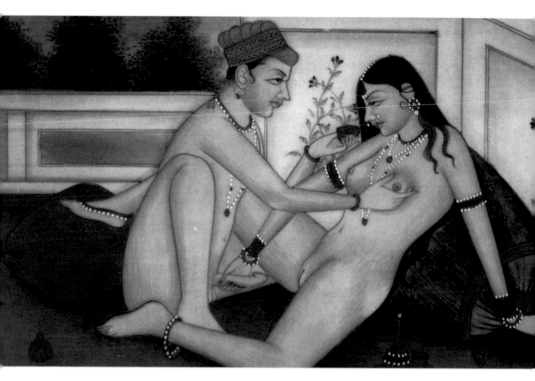

You can only give love to someone who feels it first, because everyone is divine, and then share it with someone else. As Osho says, "You cannot be in love with one person and not others. If you feel love, you feel it 24 hours a day for all beings." And we believe that we should only love one person! Obviously, your partner is your special love, a unity, but that does not stop you from loving more people. Stop your mind right away because I know you will say, Can I love the entire world, make love with the entire world? The answer is yes, but understand one thing: when you

give love (not only through sex, as there are many ways to give love), you grow, you expand. Otherwise, the light only goes in one direction. You will lose the horizon if you only look at the floor; you'll miss the valley if you're only on the mountain. Loving many people does not necessarily mean to have sex; you can love your woman or your man, obviously, by including sex in your relationship, while loving others through friendship, without sex, with sweetness and joy.

With the power of love, the feeling of existential loneliness disappears. You are not alone as you share the divinity in all beings. Remember that there is a single mother, a single parent, a single Shakti, one Shiva, a special person who accompanies you on your journey; this does not mean that you cannot love the

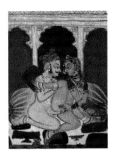

entire world. I see many couples who have enormous jealousy, which is the result of possession and the fear of losing the other. I also had to go through this, but there comes a day when you realize that you are a great lover and you have no need to be jealous because you are sure that your love will return to you every day. Many years ago I wrote a notebook's worth of notes: "Love takes you to the kingdom of heaven; possession, into the realm of jealousy." The ego feels jealousy, since love is expansive, it delights itself. And this is the sacred work that everyone should do; debug, kill the voice of the ego, and let the soul fly.

## The circuit of sexual positions

One of the most intense ways to show love, desire, and attraction is through sexual intercourse. In Tantra, when two (or more) bodies

come together, they find an internal unity. This idea changes the attitude completely; you no longer have to seek simple pleasure. The result is joy, ecstasy, pleasure, and delight. But it is also the opportunity to achieve the most intense spiritual illumination on Earth because it is meditation that mobilizes energy, flooding the brain with hormones that make it dance with the organs, which ignites the soul . . . .

It is therefore essential to know that every sexual position is a different way of circulating energy to the head, the crown chakra, the realm of Shiva, from the sexual area, the abode of kundalini shakti, the energy of life. This is the purpose of varying sexual positions and being aware of your breathing, feelings, what is inside, awakened . . . .

**One of the most intense ways to show love, desire, and attraction is through sexual intercourse.**

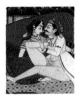

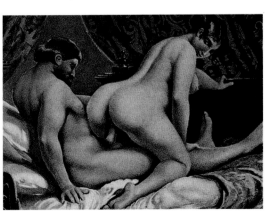

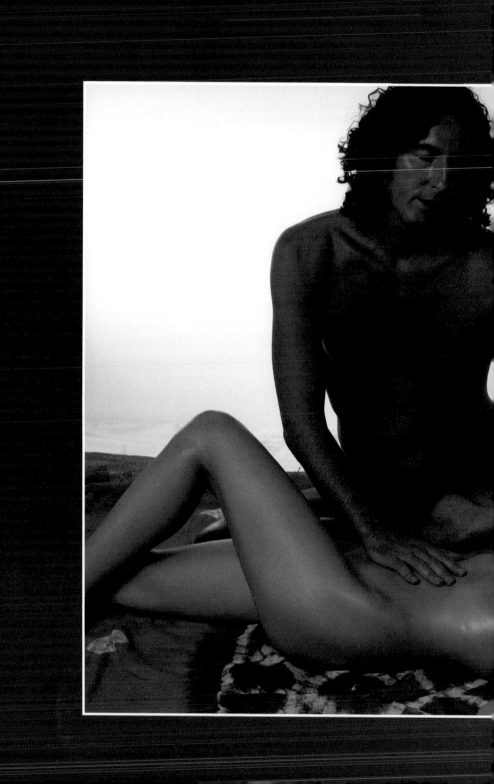

# The circuit of sexual positions

*"Every sexual position aims to build on the momentum, desire, and essentially the exchange of energy through the chakras to produce the fusion of spiritual unity between the poles."*

GUILLERMO FERRARA

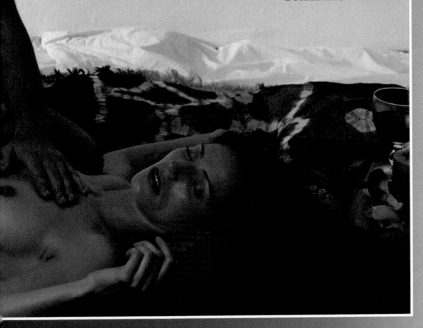

One of the most intense ways to show love, desire, and attraction is through sexual intercourse. For Tantra, when two (or more) bodies come together they find an internal unity. This idea changes the attitude completely; you no longer have to seek simple pleasure. The result is joy, ecstasy, pleasure, and delight, but is the opportunity to achieve the most intense spiritual illumination on Earth because it is meditation that mobilizes energy, flooding the brain with hormones that makes the organs dance, which ignites the soul . . . .

It is therefore essential to know that every sexual position is a different way of circulating energy to the head, the crown chakra, the realm of Shiva, from the sexual area, the abode of kundalini shakti, the energy of life. This is the purpose of varying sexual positions and to be aware of your breathing, feelings, what is inside, awakened . . . .

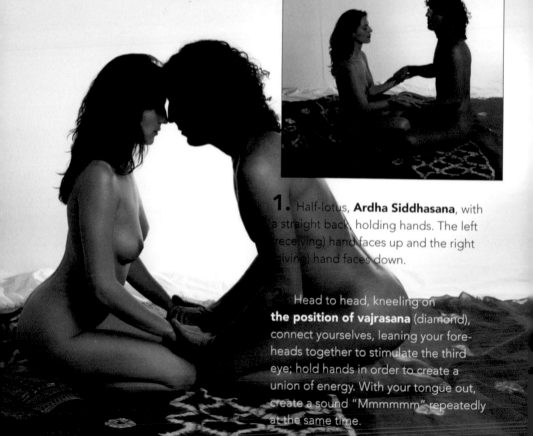

**1.** Half-lotus, **Ardha Siddhasana**, with a straight back, holding hands. The left (receiving) hand faces up and the right (giving) hand faces down.

Head to head, kneeling on **the position of vajrasana** (diamond), connect yourselves, leaning your foreheads together to stimulate the third eye; hold hands in order to create a union of energy. With your tongue out, create a sound "Mmmmmm" repeatedly at the same time.

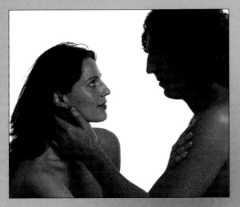

**3.** Begin to **stimulate yourself by caressing** all of your body while you look each other in the eye. This starts to increase your desire.

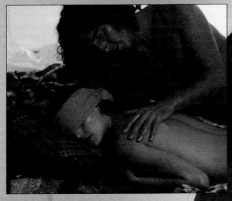

**4. Stimulate through touch**, star[ting] in the back and moving to the fron[t.] Touch your lover's body in a loving [and] subtle way. Use a blindfold to feel [it] more deeply.

**5.** Give the **"Kiss of Life"** to each other, with the ver[s]ation of sex through your mouth (oral se[x]. First do it individ-ually and then togeth[er] at the same time in the c[re]w position [or through] "69." Tantra m[  ] [en]ergetic currents emitted [by] sex [  ] a [  ] form al[ng] with [  ]o gre[  ] pleasure.

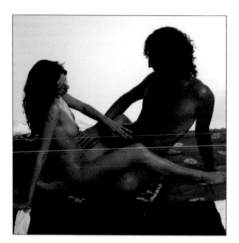

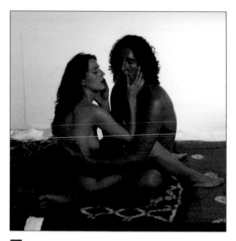

**6.** **Awaken the erotic points of the navel by making circles**, changing the pressure from hard to soft. Awakening the navel brings about even more sexual energy.

**7.** Do the same with **your fingers in his mouth**, playing with his lips, sucking the fingers of your lover. The mouth is directly tied to sex.

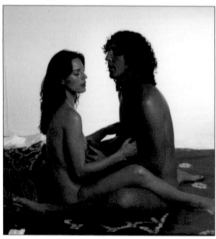

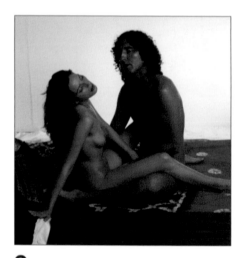

**8.** **Activate the energy in the nipples**, touching them gently, squeezing them, playing with them, making circles. This enhances the positive pole in women and the negative pole in men; it carries sexual energy through the rest of the body.

**9.** **Sexual stroking**. The woman plays with the lungam (the shaft and the glans) and the testes, pressing softly first and then more intensely. The man touches, like a feather, the clitoris, labia, pubic hair (which should be as bulky and natural as Kali) and then the G-spot (the "crown jewel").

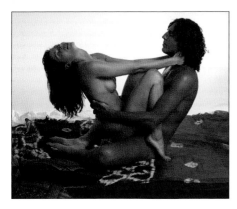

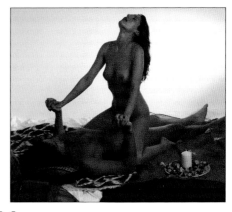

**10.** **The swing**. Shiva sits with the souls of her feet together while receiving Shakti, which goes on with his legs apart and folded against his chest. He holds Shiva's neck. If the desire is intense enough, he can penetrate her. Enjoy this first contact, feeling the slow penetration.

**11.** **The mare**. After several minutes, Shiva sits back against Shakti. While holding hands, let his desire increase. The man should practice a slow breath and relax his whole body, "letting him love himself."

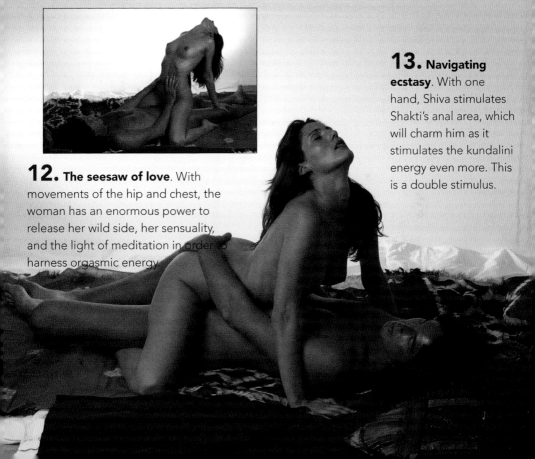

**13.** **Navigating ecstasy**. With one hand, Shiva stimulates Shakti's anal area, which will charm him as it stimulates the kundalini energy even more. This is a double stimulus.

**12.** **The seesaw of love**. With movements of the hip and chest, the woman has an enormous power to release her wild side, her sensuality, and the light of meditation in order to harness orgasmic energy.

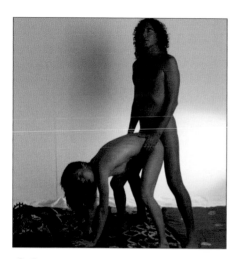

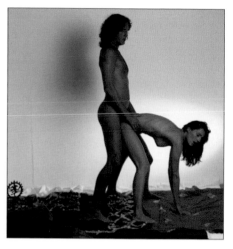

**14.** **The elephant pose** or **the union of the cow**. The woman opens her legs and bends forward with her hands on the floor. The man, standing in back, makes circular motions while penetrating, alternating forward and backwards movements while breathing deeply. When he inhales, he goes forward (to take in the energy of the yoni) and when he goes backwards he exhales.

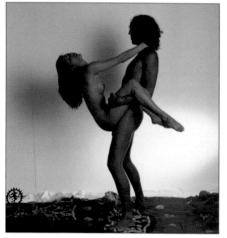

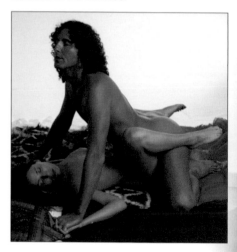

**15.** **The suspended union or the big jump**. Shiva argues with Shakti with his hands clasped on her thighs. She forcefully holds his neck. He demonstrates his power with circular motions.

**16.** **The crab** or **a very open stance**. Shakti lies down with her legs open and Shiva penetrates her with different depths while holding hands so the chakras can connect even more.

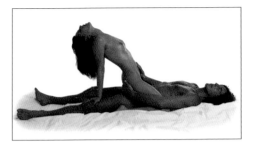

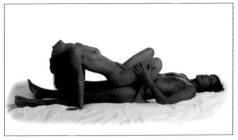

**17.** Now you will change roles, **going back and forth** with love. Shiva becomes passive and Shakti climbs on with bent legs, breathing deeply as to bring about the orgasmic energy from the brain to the rest of the body.

**18.** **The boat**. By varying the position of open legs resting on the floor, Shakti secures her hands backwards so that they open on his chest. This allows a release of the forward chakras. Shiva, at the same time she is being penetrated, can gently stimulate her clitoris.

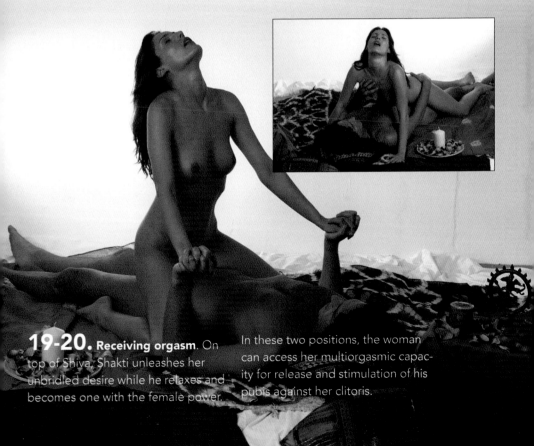

**19-20.** **Receiving orgasm**. On top of Shiva, Shakti unleashes her unbridled desire while he relaxes and becomes one with the female power. In these two positions, the woman can access her multiorgasmic capacity for release and stimulation of his pubis against her clitoris.

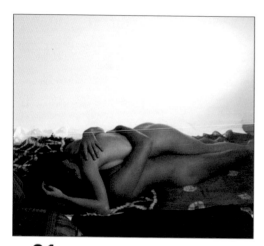

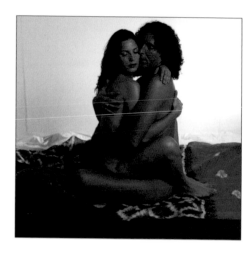

**21.** **Fusion of the chakras.** Leaning over him, Shakti harmonizes her breathing (which at this time should be like a locomotive) in order to synchronize and channel a sexual fire.

**22.** **The yab-yum.** Meditate in an almost immobile state connecting Muladhara to Sahasrara chakras.

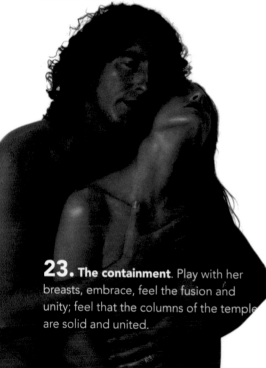

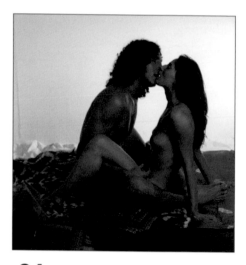

**23.** **The containment.** Play with her breasts, embrace, feel the fusion and unity; feel that the columns of the temple are solid and united.

**24.** **Resuming desire.** Stimulate each other with a variety of kisses that Tantra proposes. Shakti is right and Shiva returns to penetrate her thighs, which allows movement and rekindles desire.

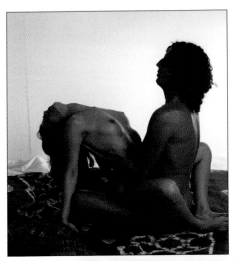

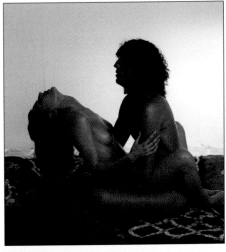

## 25-26-27. Circular motion.

Shakti above Shiva, in the Yab-Yum, will move forward and backward, with intense breathing. When you move forward, inhale the exhaled air of Shiva, his breath of life. The energetic currents produced by combining movement and breath are very intense.

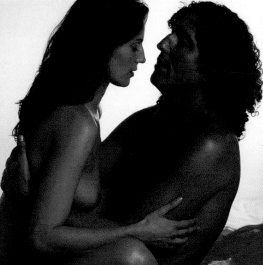

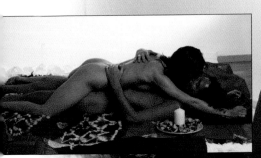

## 28. Shared union.

Shakti lies above Shiva, joining from the sexual area, the mouth and the chakras. She can stay motionless, meditating on shared power, and move alternately so that the pubis and clitoris are both stimulated.

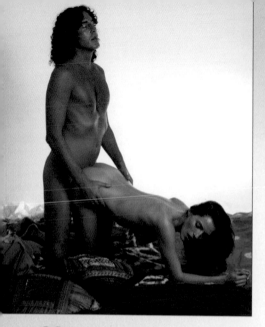

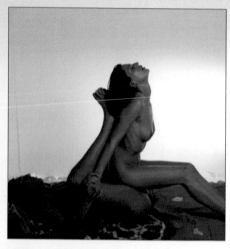

## 29. The tiger attacks from behind.

The woman, with her knees and elbows supported, lets the man penetrate from behind. Shiva alternates movements forward and backward (remember to inhale as you move forward and exhale as you move back, as upon exhaling one is more likely to ejaculate) and also in circular movements. Vary the intensity, ranging from smooth and slow to intense, strong, and deep.

## 30. Swivel posture.

The man reclines with his legs half bent and the woman takes all of his lingam and leans back on her legs. This penetration is very intense and stimulates the female G-Spot.

**The delivery.** Shakti lays on her back on the breast of Shiva, who continues penetration and caresses her entire body, with an emphasis on breasts, nipples, navel, pubic, armpits, and clitoris. Here the man can feel an orgasm without ejaculation (breathing and letting his desire rise) by the intense fire that vibrates in his body and that of his beloved.

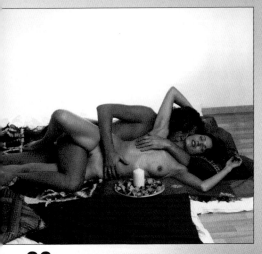

**32. Lateral posture**. Shakti lies on one side and Shiva stands behind, penetrating her softly. A woman loves being taken from behind, as it arouses great devotion and protection.

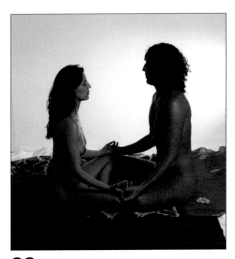

**33. Shared meditation**. Every 30 or 40 minutes during positions in rotation, Tantra recommends meditating on your shared energy. In the half-lotus, sitting face to face, channel the fire of sexual chakras.

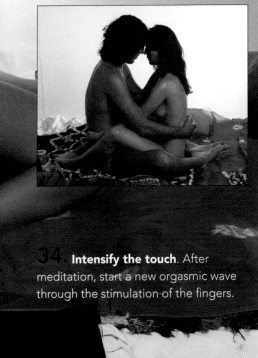

34. **Intensify the touch**. After meditation, start a new orgasmic wave through the stimulation of the fingers.

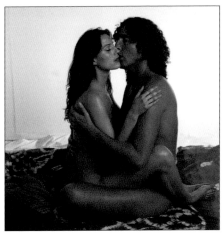

**35. Kissing, touching, and smelling**. Combine these three senses in order for electricity to rise to a new wave (you can make the climb/excitement, and descent/relaxation, as often as you feel).

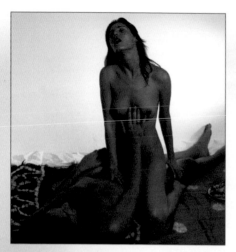

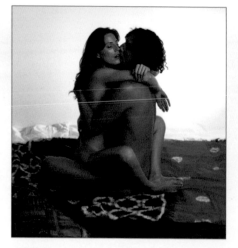

**36.** **Kali**. The woman has her legs bent and feet flat on the floor. With intense, wild, and free movements, Shakti lets the power of the goddess Kali seize her, transforming her into an incandescent flame of passion and decauchery. This is a test of fire for men. Relax your body, go down with one hand down to your testicles so there is no tension and you will enjoy har- mony with your woman.

**37.** **The eternal embrace.** Sitting face to face with an intense union of desire, seal your encounter with a hug that goes from strong to soft. Hug and maintain immobile penetration. This gives lovers one of the most sublime experiences on this planet: feeling the woman and man in full androgy- nous communion. When vibrating correctly, the mind transcends the two bodies and becomes one while our souls fly free into a sky of expanded consciousness.

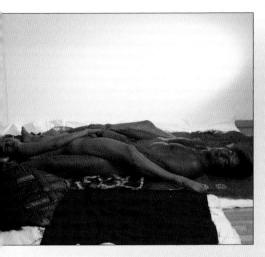

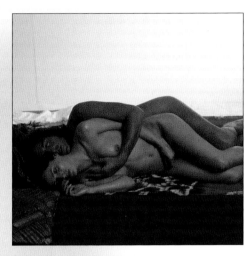

**39.** **The X position**. While penetrated with open legs and leaning backwards, take each other's hands and dive into the yoga nidra. Feel the Buddha state when everything vibrates in the light and is a vast ocean of bliss. Here is where relaxation, meditation, and "the valley of orgasm," which appears as an infinite state of peace, connection, fulfillment, company, fusion, quietness, sweetness, love, and delight, all begin.

**40.** **The spoon**. Sleep on the opposite side of the heart—Shiva behind Shakti, or vice versa—so that the currents that are generated perform in a more subtle and unconscious level. Often, the energy that has been shared and accumulated allows for entry to the astral planes, where advanced tantric initiations by teachers, goddesses, and other devas are made. This is for the disciplined candidates and a more advanced chapter. Practice these circuits, and one day they will come to you . . . .

**38.** **Fusion of the Chakras**. Looking for relaxation, the woman lies on top of a relaxed man and shares pleasurable kisses and appreciated caresses.

The *Kama Sutra* [...] at in order to fill [...] different insight [...] do not settle for le[...]

1. **Thrust forward.** When the organs are [...] ly and directly
2. **Friction.** He holds the lingam with h[...] the yoni.
3. **The lingam penetrates to the bo[...]**
4. **Blows.** It is as in the previous case, [...] the [...] us the bottom of the yoni.
5. **Pre[...]s.** The yoni comes in con[...] gam for a long time and altern[...]ely with the "secret langua[...] ax and vice versa
6. **Sl[...]ing.** The lingam is removed [...] with great force into the yo[...]
7. **W[...]boar attack.** The lingam just [...] the yoni.
8. **B[...]ttack.** Both sides of the yoni [...] lingam
9. **[...]t of the sparrow.** The lingam [...] rapidly without ta[...] [b]reak. This act can terminate the co[...]

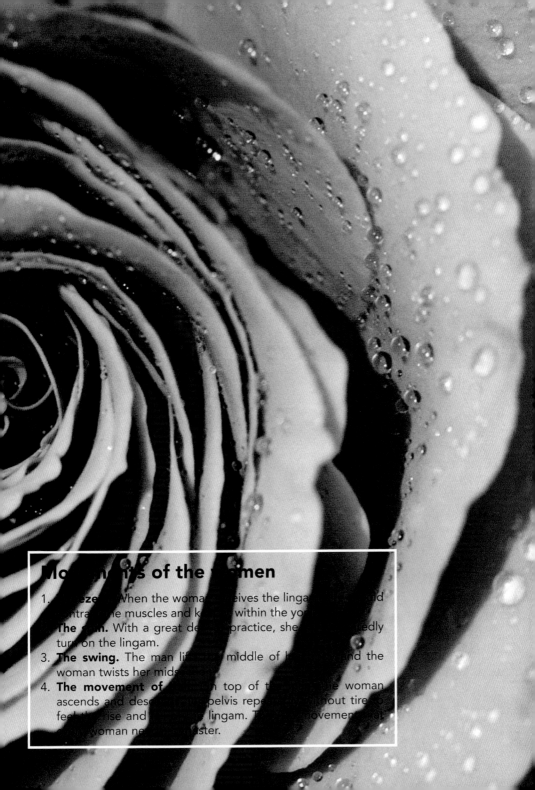

## Movements of the women

1. **Squeeze.** When the woman receives the lingam she should contract the muscles and keep it within the yoni.
2. **The spin.** With a great deal of practice, she can repeatedly turn on the lingam.
3. **The swing.** The man lifts the middle of his body and the woman twists her midsection.
4. **The movement of** when on top of the man, the woman ascends and descends her pelvis repeatedly without tiring to feel the rise and fall of the lingam. This is a movement that every woman needs to master.

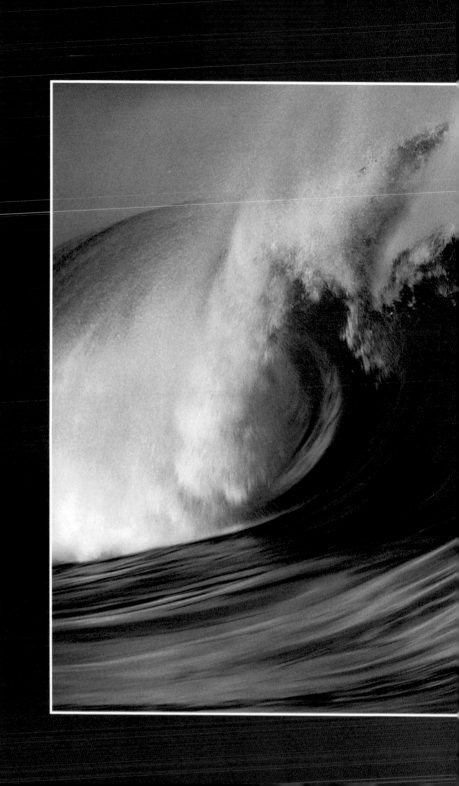

# Ejaculation and orgasm

*"Tantra seeks to redirect energy and open a wedge to the divine through orgasm."*

GUILLERMO FERRARA

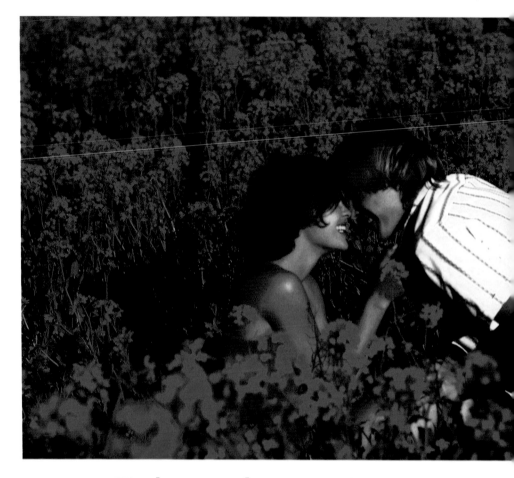

# To know the tantric orgasm is to enter paradise

**In the beginning, we lived in a state of paradise.**

In the beginning, we lived in a state of paradise, in awe, latent, orgasmic, with the instinct to surface. He who says that God said "Thou shalt not eat the fruit" forgets that he meant not to waste sexual energy through ejaculation, not a simple apple, since ejaculation lowers the life energy of kundalini Shakti from the crown chakra (where spiritual awareness is opened) to the muladhara chakra (in the lower area, the animal instinct).

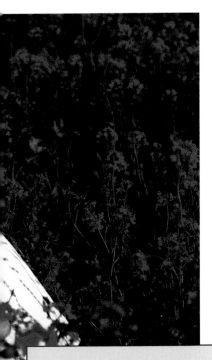

Thus, if a person maintains his vital oil and rises upwards, he will live in a state of expanded consciousness in the ecstasy that arises from the supreme connection. This connection is our ultimate legacy and flows through our interior naturally before the ideas of the mind, taboos, and fears of the naturalness of sexual energy poison us.

Tantra seeks to redirect this energy and drive a wedge into the divine through orgasm. At that moment, the feeling of cosmic expansion is like an atomic explosion, like an internal atomic bomb

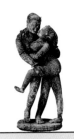

# Déjà vu, remember your origin?

When sexual energy is transformed, many internal powers begin to awaken, which shows that we already have them, but they are asleep. For example, the feeling that you've had an experience or have been to a place before is known as déjà vu ("already seen" in French). In Tantra, you learn to see mental images as if film is involved.

This is the aim of the sexual sculptures carved in stone in the temple of Khajuraho in India. These sculptures are there in order to show all possible ways to perform the sexual act so that once seen, we are left to fantasize about them. Inside the temple, however, it is empty; there are no images or symbols. Similarly, to perform various sexual positions, the mind of the tantric partner is satisfied and full, and then enter the inner emptiness, the peace and delight of satisfied desire. When you encounter déjà vu, look closely so you can communicate with that experience; maybe you can learn something from it. If, for example, you perform mirror meditation (carefully observing your own face), it will start to distort after a while; Tantra says that you can now see the face of your previous life.

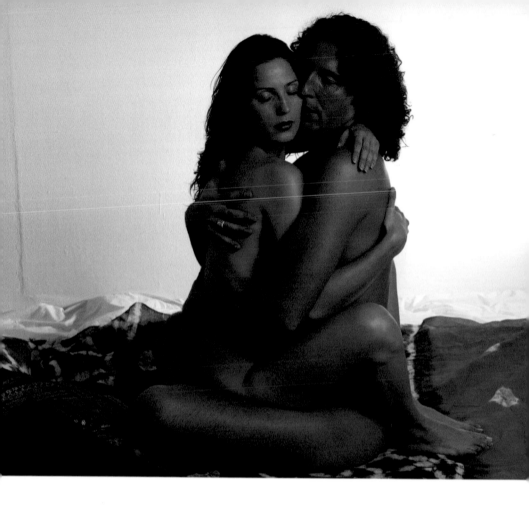

**Sometimes a hug creates a sense of profound unity even though two people are strangers.**

where electricity and vitality dispel the internal limits. This does not happen if there are repeated ejaculations or if sex is used as a release of tension. This is simply a waste of vital energy, a slow death, not a transformation of the inner alchemy that everyone should manifest in their bodies.

Therefore, for the tantric practitioner, it may feel like that Paradise is a state of consciousness and not a specific place.

## The tantric embrace

Shiva says, "When in such an embrace, your senses shake like leaves, remaining in him."

Sometimes a hug creates a profound sense of unity, even if two people are strangers. Hugging is the fusion of both energies in one, it is the momentary victory over solitude, the delight of feeling the other as oneself. Hugging is also a way to connect the chakras since the seven engage with the energy of the other. For example, the position of Yab-Yum, wherein Shakti sits astride Shiva, is the ideal place to feel the supreme, long hug. If penetration happens in this position, it's even better, but you will feel that connection.

A hug requires delivery, the heart opens. Delve into the embrace as if you are a vine that is woven into the body and soul of another; every hug whispers a secret in its own language.

In the sexual maithuna, the embrace in the Yab-Yum position accompanies swaying bodies that enable, through movement, waves of ecstasy into conscious and internal expansion.

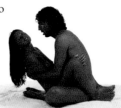

**"When in such an embrace, your senses shake like leaves, remaining in him."**

## Watch out: the avalanche!

When you're making so much energy, orgasms succeed each other in a matter of minutes. When you know the rhythms and explore the body of your loved one or your beloved, you know which trigger points and positions create orgasms. When Shakti and Shiva are lying and she is on top of him, she should stimulate his anus with her middle finger while he penetrates with the lingam. This causes the kundalini energy to awaken and ascends even more. On the other hand, if one wants to feel the orgasm of his companion, this area will feel ten to twenty orgasmic contractions. This is precisely the moment when Shakti—dynamic, explosive, natural, wild, and sensitive— begins to awaken. It is a shame that for many people, this is the end of the sexual experience, when Taoism mentions that unless a female receives three thousand lingam movements (in and out), she will not be satiated.

It is not necesary to obsess about the number of movements, but know that it is important to have plenty of time to go into much deeper states, as sexual energy will be like an avalanche that provides heavy and successive waves.

A woman can have many orgasms in a sexual act (that is the natural right of the female gender) and a man can feel an orgasm without ejaculating by boosting his sexual energy and storing it without discharging it outside.

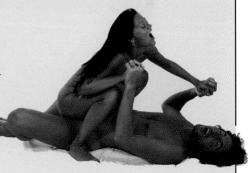

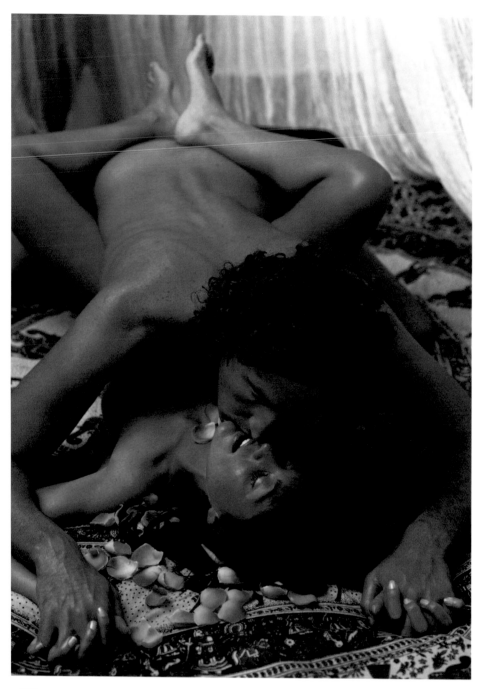

# Increase your desire

The secret to the sexual act is the prolongation of desire. With ejaculation, desire ends. The magic disappears, vanishes, and you feel a disconnection. It momentarily relieves tensions, but the couple is found light years away from each other.

With a permanent desire, you have sexual energy the entire time; you always want to have sex because you are alive, glowing, and you should be. There is no need to wait for a special moment or something to light the spark; our bodies are sexual; thousands and thousands of trillions of our cells are sexual, and their cores are light. If you live with fear or you cover your entire body, this light is shut off.

The tantric practice turns on the lights in each of your cells; they are vital, healthy, and radiant again. Every time a thought of lack, fear, or insecurity runs through the theater of the mind, the cells are off for a while. If the desire is on, there

is life itself in its present essence, because the origin of life is desire. In India, Earth is called *Kama Loka* or "world of desires." The sexual desire for unity is the basic desire of the human species. Not that there are no other desires; there are seven basic desires in every individual, but if the desire for life is repressed, other obstacles and blockages will occur in other areas.

With meditation of the androgynous, that is to touch the body in order to activate the kundalini, the latent desire will always be awake and ready to be shared.

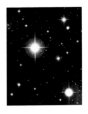

**Thousands and thousands of trillions of our cells are sexual, and their cores are light.**

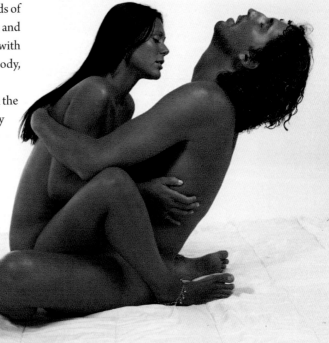

# Sexual secrets of the tantric orgasm

Let's learn the sexual secrets of the tantric orgasm. Certain pre-maithuna practices exist that everyone must exercise alone in order to dominate this energy when entering into ritual practices.

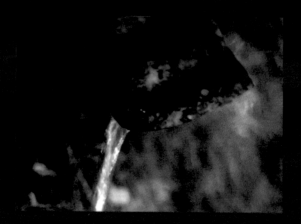

## 1. URINARY TRACT

Each time you go to make a small pee, make short contractions of the uniary muscles, the pubococcygeus; this way you will strengthen the muscles responsible for ejaculation in men and enhance orgasms and sensations in women.

## 2. SPECIAL BREATHING

When you are very excited, use kapalabhati or bhastrika breathing. Breathe through your nose alternately and quickly, feeling the solar plexus with each breath. After twenty dynamic breaths, you will, from time to time, create even more energy and decentralize the sexual area. A tantric lover delights to hear the breath of his counterpart.

Make complete, slow, deep breaths and you will feel that desire will continue and expands consciousness.

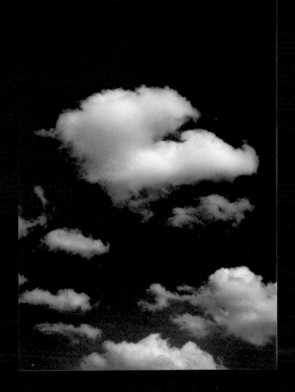

## 3. ASVINI MUDRA

You can always do this exercise, which depends on the retention of ejaculation.

Contract and loosen the pubococcygeus muscle quickly throughout the day while standing or sitting. This will also generate *tummo* or internal heat. With this exercise, naked Tibetan llamas dry the clothes wrapped around them when they are wet. If this is true, it would be much easier to carry the laundry. This *kriya* is used to get to know the internal heat, the meandering fire in our body, and to enhance it.

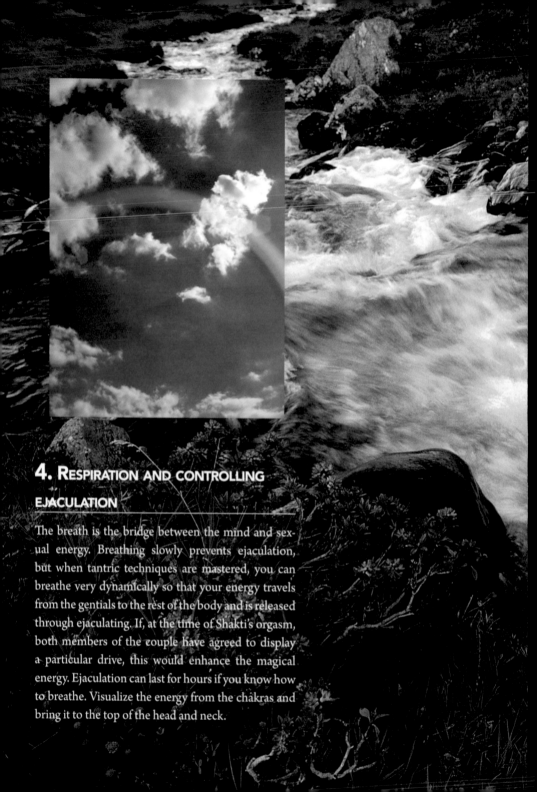

## 4. Respiration and Controlling

### Ejaculation

The breath is the bridge between the mind and sexual energy. Breathing slowly prevents ejaculation, but when tantric techniques are mastered, you can breathe very dynamically so that your energy travels from the gentials to the rest of the body and is released through ejaculating. If, at the time of Shakti's orgasm, both members of the couple have agreed to display a particular drive, this would enhance the magical energy. Ejaculation can last for hours if you know how to breathe. Visualize the energy from the chakras and bring it to the top of the head and neck.

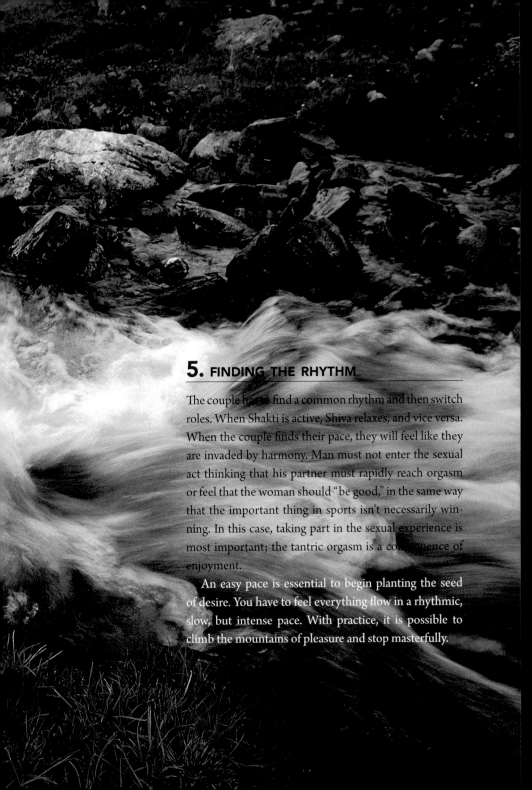

## 5. FINDING THE RHYTHM

The couple has to find a common rhythm and then switch roles. When Shakti is active, Shiva relaxes, and vice versa. When the couple finds their pace, they will feel like they are invaded by harmony. Man must not enter the sexual act thinking that his partner must rapidly reach orgasm or feel that the woman should "be good," in the same way that the important thing in sports isn't necessarily winning. In this case, taking part in the sexual experience is most important; the tantric orgasm is a consequence of enjoyment.

An easy pace is essential to begin planting the seed of desire. You have to feel everything flow in a rhythmic, slow, but intense pace. With practice, it is possible to climb the mountains of pleasure and stop masterfully.

## THE TESTICLES

...breathe and channel energy through his body. When the voltage of the testicles has disappeared, the urge to ejaculate will too.

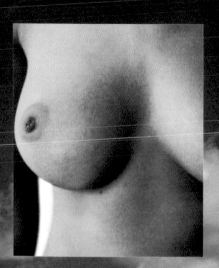

## 7. THE NIPPLES

The sexual organs are positive in men and negative in women.

When two bodies meet, their energy bars are attached in the same way as electricity; you have to encourage each other to make good contact with the opposite pole of energy. This must be done gently with time to awaken the yoni and the lingam.

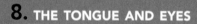

## 8. THE TONGUE AND EYES

Bringing the tongue back and keeping the eyes closed is also a good technique to increase energy. Stop upon arriving at the summit and make this *kriya*.

## 9. SIRSASANA

The position (asana) of the yogic head stand is an advanced form of Tantra (Tantric Yoga) that is extremely benefical to bring energy to the brain. However, we should do this asana without having practiced yoga for at least 3 months.

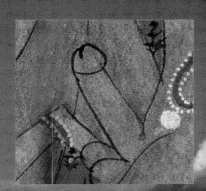

## 10. THE GLANS

The glans is a highly sensitive and energetic area. Shakti has to learn to play with the glans and stimulate it as if it were her own; she can travel over it with her mouth or with her fingers, as this delights Shiva. She can also wrap her hand around it and squeeze it gently to stop ejaculation.

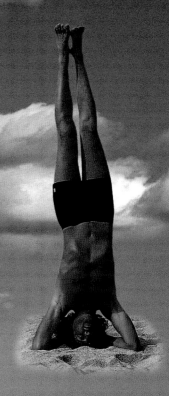

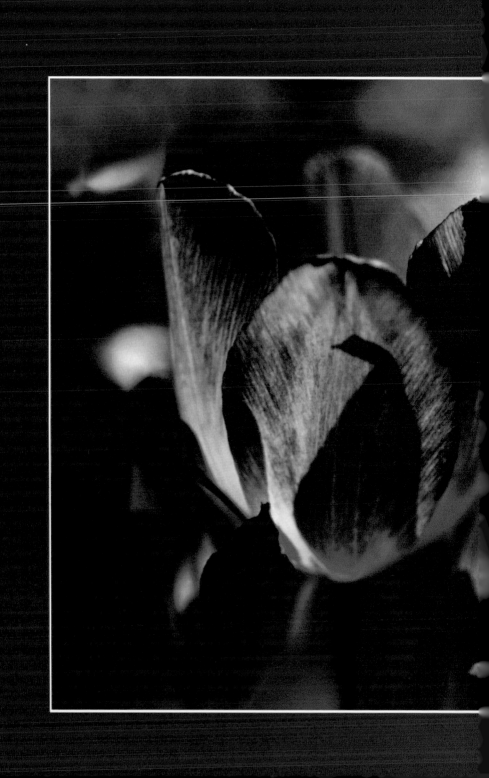

# Lessons in tantric sex

*Tantra is the supreme wisdom, in all the arts of life, and the act that gives it is sex. Through sex you know life.*

GUILLERMO FERRARA

## Lesson 1

# Shiva and Shakti: consciousness and energy

As we have been saying through this book, for Tantra, each woman, in her deepest essence, is **Shakti**, and each man is **Shiva**. The sacredness of everyone unites us together and transcends personality, time, death, and being. Each individual also has an ego, often away from the essence, troubled by the voices of the mind and personal selfishness. The ego is full of jealousy, fears, traumas, etc. With practice, Tantra absorbs us into our true identity that is light, openness, expansion, creativity, fluidity, and loveliness. The change is to allow our consciousness to become one with Shiva and Shakti. We will take this first lesson to affirm our experiences.

## Note:

Practice each lesson for an entire day. If you are together in the morning, you can determine which practices you are going to do all day. Practice at your own pace and pay attention to the results. The order here is not necessarily an established order, but can serve as a guide to achieve mastery.

**1.** Repeat the following affirmatio as many times during the day as you choose. The statements are then recorded in the subconscious, which is a receptacle that responds to wha we put into it, so in this way we can prepare our consciousness. With thi statement, you will initiate the ritual Shiva and Shakti. "I am light, I am a eternal being. I am the dance of life I am the sun and the moon, I am the fusion of the original energy."

**2.** Having prepared the ritual plac for food and drink, with candles anc incense, say, "I present the nakednes of my body and soul." Here you will look at your partner's body in order increase your own sense of sight an to ponder the beauty of the body.

**3.** Holding hands, begin to chant the mantra *Om namah shivaia*. Ther hum *Om shakti*. Do this seven times for each.

**4.** Shakti will perform a sensual dance and Shiva will do the same. Move the entire body so that the

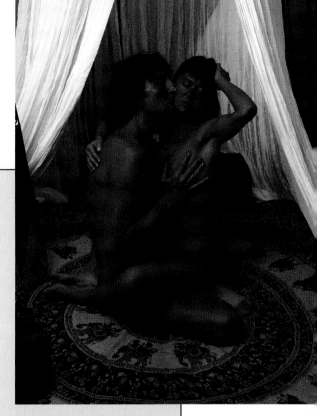

movement begins to mobilize energy; express yourself, seduce, and eroticize. Then hold hands and dance together.

**5.** With your backs touching, sit in a meditative posture while your connected chakras merge both heat and vibration; do this for fifteen minutes. Take your hands and connect yourselves with the sacrum; put them behind your backs and touch.

**6.** Sitting face to face, take your hands and place them on your foreheads. Breathe in unison for a few minutes in order to feel the same breath. Alternate and cycle the air so Shakti inhales while Shiva exhales. Change the prana to provide a fusion of communication and life energy.

**7.** Use oil on your bodies and activate all of the different sensations. Touch each other gently, sensually, and with connection. Let the first language of humanity, touch, be expressed beyond the limits of the mind. Touch, feel, breathe, and delight in order to take you to the heights of joy, awareness, and energetic rapport.

**Finale.** After the ritual, lay down and relax while meditating and sharing power in silence. Preserve the electric charge that was generated, accumulating desire without sexual intercourse. Keep this engraved in your hearts with intense burning. Share peace, food, and drink in honor of Shiva and Shakti and save your maithuna for another day.

## Lesson 2

# The yab-yum

The yab-yum is the most recommended tantric sexual position. The woman positions herself above the man with open legs. Both sit with their spines straightened and Shiva crosses his legs in a half lotus.

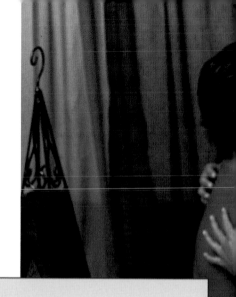

**1.** In the yab-yum position (without penetration), think about your lover's breathing. Each time Shakti exhales, Shiva breathes in through the nostrils, and vice versa. Do this for fifteen minutes. This will produce an important alchemy of energy in addition to focusing attention on the energies of both people.

**2.** Keeping the tongue on the palate and the mouth closed, repeat the sound "mmmmmm" with each exhalation. This sound will produce an awakening of the pineal gland and the ajna chakra, the third eye.

**3.** Activate your kundalini energy by touching erotic points of the body: mouth, neck, nipples, armpits, hands, navel, genitals, thighs, toes . . .

**4.** Next, revive the sinuous sexual fire through the five forms of kissing: blows, bites, suction of the lips, kissing with the tongue, and lip kissing. The contact of the tongue awakens sexual energies through the central sushumna channel.

**5.** Make love in the Yab-Yum position freely, letting the soft cadence enter you into a deep meditative state while allowing physical pleasure to invade. Utilize this position only to enhance the chakras. This is highly recommended for anyone who is just starting as it helps control ejaculation.

**6.** When finished, lie down one after another on the right side (opposite the heart), maintaining contact with the back and chest, and stay deeply relaxed.

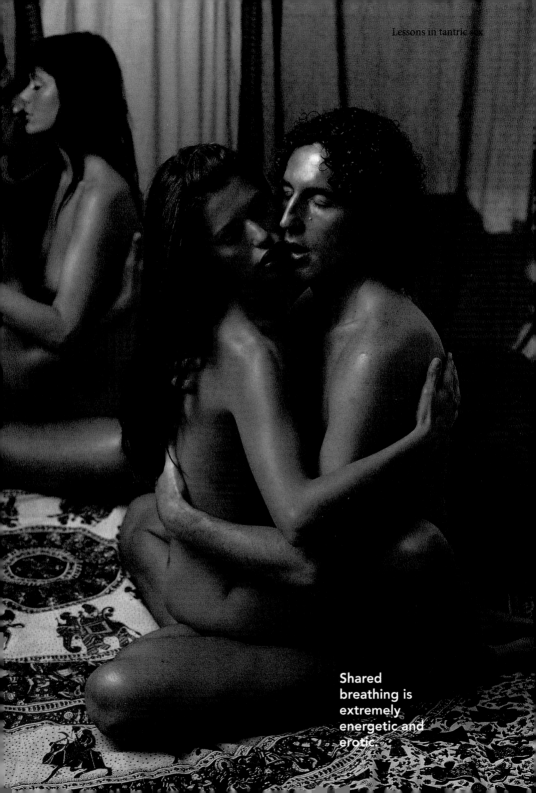

Shared
breathing is
extremely
energetic and
erotic.

## Lesson 3

# Energy

Vital energy is a phenomenon that produces life and movement. The *prana* is what comes out of the sun and through breathing, air is the vehicle that starts our body and all life on the planet. We also receive energy from the earth, the *apana*. This lesson serves to increase the vital energy every day.

**1.** Standing naked, shake your body from head to toe. Do this for ten minutes while you breathe deeply through your nose, dynamic and short, like a bellows. This will fully recharge the energy system and chakras by combining movement and breath. Do this in front of a window for fresh air.

**2.** Sitting motionless in a meditative posture, take in complete breaths and visualize breathing a column of fire in order to increase your energy.

**3.** Produce three bolts or bhandas: Mulhadara bandha by contracting the buttocks and anus; Uddiyana bandha by raising the abdomen and sinking the navel; and the Jalandhara bandha by placing your chin into your chest and engaging in a throat or chin "lock." Retain the air for 8 to 10 seconds and repeat 7 times. Visualize the energy as golden oil that runs through the nose or meridians as if they were veins of fire or "rivers of living water."

**4.** Give yourself to practicing abdominal breathing: do this so that the abdomen swells and exhales, letting out the air.

**5.** Assemble your hands on your chest, gradually separating your palms five, ten, and fifteen centimeters apart. You will feel a tingling sensation in both hands. Do this alone first and then with your partner.

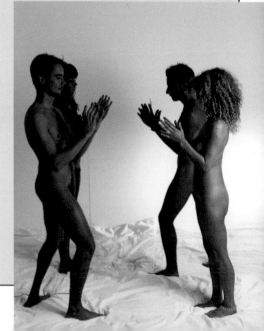

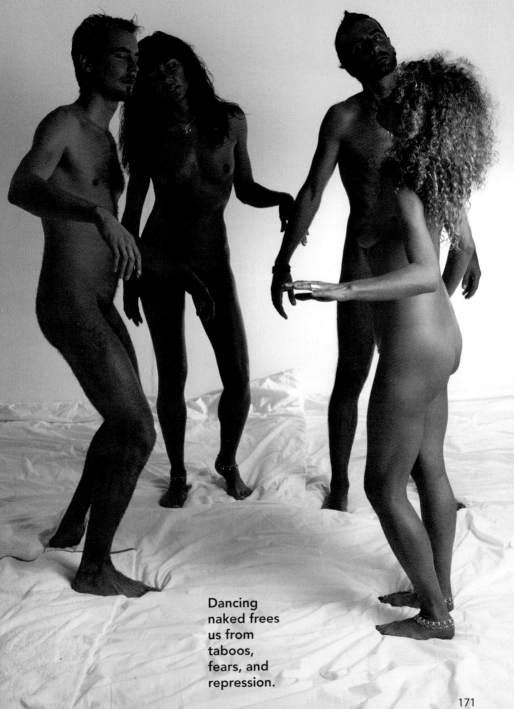

Dancing
naked frees
us from
taboos,
fears, and
repression.

Lesson 4

# The art of the body

The body is a sacred temple and is revered because it is a divine gift. We attend and care for the body from all angles, not to mention the soul.

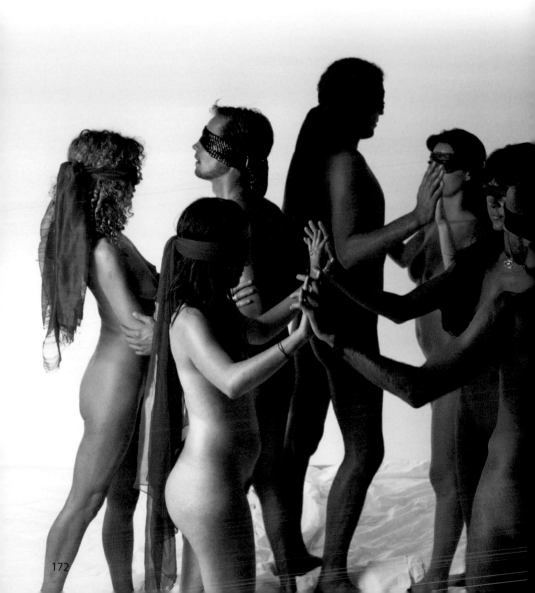

**1.** Observe the beauty of your partner's naked body or of the other couples who join you to practice Tantra.

**2.** Spread sweet almond oil with jasmine, sandalwood, or musk, and feel that each body part encompasses the whole. Concentrate on each appendage and the service it provides, starting with the feet and ending with the head.

**3.** Continue across your lover's body, feeling the energy in your fingertips. Vary the pressure. Go from a touch as soft as a feather to one of maximum intensity. If you include another tantric couple, share among

everyone, leaving communication to intellect and feeling through body language, your inner voice, so you can be filled with pleasure and relaxation. This is the formula to disintegrate mental poisons. Do this for at least thirty minutes, consciously inspiring energy that emerges from your bodies. You will be pure fire, attraction, energy, and consciousness.

**4.** Cover your eyes, and if you do this with one or more partner, seek your love through touch.

**5.** Without using your hands, establish contact with each other's bodies through the chest, back, shoulders, and legs, triggering friction.

**6.** Continue touching with devotion and softness from the toes to the head and enter a deep state of relaxation.

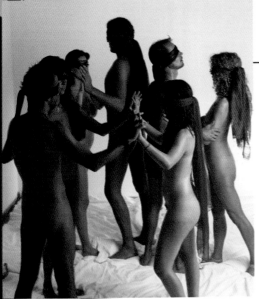

**Touching is the bridge that unites practitioners beyond the mind.**

## Lesson 5

# Emotions and thoughts

**Releasing anger gives way to inner peace.**

"Emotion" means "moving energy from inside to the outside." When you suppress an emotion, you are blocking the creative energy of life. We are emotional beings—aquatic, not terrestrial. Life is pure emotion. Expressing emotion means letting the heart speak. Emotions are the voice of the heart and thoughts of the mind. We often repress our feelings with thoughts of fear, anger, or concern. The heart is brave; it is in direct connection with the great heart that is God. The formula of Tantra is to unite intelligence and heart...for love is not blind, but prescient! My first teacher taught me, "Wisdom is knowing what you feel and feeling what you know."

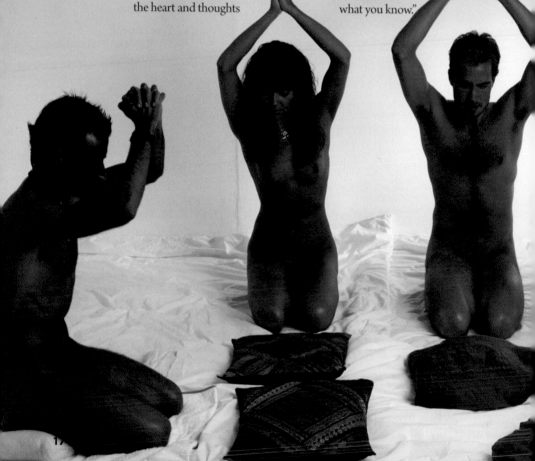

**1.** Make a list of how you express the following emotions:

**Anger**. Do you show it or repress it?
**Fear**. Does it dominate you or do you confront it?
**Worry**. Are you worried about something most of the time?
**Guilt**. Do you feel guilty about something? Is this something real or something you invented?
**Boredom**. Do you feel like you are sick of some person, thing, or activity?

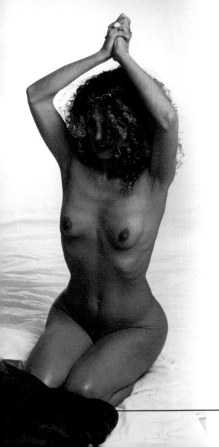

**2.** To discharge anger, take a pillow and beat it against the ground as many times as you need until you feel relaxed. You can also do the exercise of the lumberjack: standing with legs apart and hands interlaced, take a breath, take your arms up, and forcefully swing them while shouting "Ah" several times.

**3.** Spend an afternoon reflecting on your emotions; this is best when done in a park or garden.

**4.** Make a list of all of the thoughts that come to mind for 3 hours.

**5.** Create gibberish: pronounce meaningless sounds as if speaking in an unknown language for ten minutes. This provides a fantastic cleaning of the parasites of mental confusion and completely renews your mental energy.

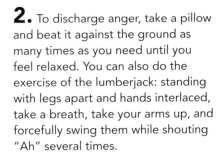

**2**

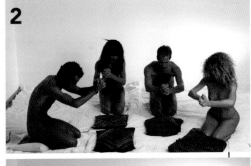

**3**

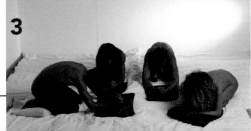

# The naked fire ritual

Inside our bodies are all of the elements; fire is the archetype of spiritual power. It is the element that goes up, ascending against gravity. The three phases of fire are spark, flame, and ember. When a person awakens the spiritual world, that world's spark connects with one's inner reality and can change one's consciousness. Humanity evolves in two ways: as a group and a species (this is an unconscious evolution through genetics, history, and experience) and individually (conscious, unique, responsible). Daydreaming about the inner fire makes the kundalini flame rise by strengthening the astral chakras, which are the basis for the human psyche.

**1.** Find a secluded place where there are no distractions.

**2.** You can invite a couple more participants.

**3.** If you want music, rhythmically play drums to enhance the experience and the sense of sound. The naked body feels open and repression will be cast into the fire.

**4.** Kindle the fire, asking permission from the superior forces with a prayer "Force of wonderful love, may the sacred fires revive in order to awaken my conscience."

In many places, it is customary to light bonfires with old furniture to celebrate the summer solstice. This ritual symbolizes the burning of old wounds or negative experiences that prevent evolution.

In each chakra there is a particular item or element. Earth corresponds to the first chakra, water to the second, fire to the third, air to the fourth, ether to the fifth, thought to the sixth, and light to the seventh.

Here we perform the ritual of naked fire. The fire was formerly revered and cared for for days, and participants kept it going with purpose, among other things, to raise awareness.

Many shamanic exercises also have to do with this purpose. In Mexico, it is a shamanic custom to stay alone in a mountain house to keep this fire burning for ten days. After this time, the conscious is clear, expanded, powerful, and full of light.

**5.** Sitting in a meditative posture, meditate on the fire while watching the flames. Repeat the mantra *Om mani padme hum* ("Oh, the divine within me") or the mantra of mantras, OM.

**6.** Stretch your hands towards the flames at a distance to feel the heat and energy through the chakras.

**7.** You can set fire to an old garment or something that represents the burning of a negative emotion of the past. You can also write a desire on the object before burning it so that the emotion becomes concrete. Meditate on this for a few minutes and then throw it in the blaze with conviction.

**8.** Meditate on the crackling flames and let its heat and sound penetrate and purify the consciousness and astral energetic field.

**9.** When you see the flames dwindle, rest yourself in order to feel the peace and fullness of the coals. Do not quench the fire with dirt or water; let it burn out.

Daydreaming about the inner fire allows the kundalini flame to ascend the astral column.

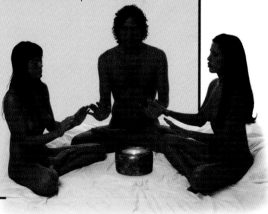

## Lesson 7

# The tantric circle

The circle is the symbol of perfection. Like the Ouroboros, the dragon that bites its tail, completing an eternal circle without beginning or ending, the tantric circle ritual allows the feeling of inner eternity that transcends the feeling of physical death. The embrace of our bodies affects the inner consciousness and makes us full lovers.

**1.** While naked, rub oil on the front of the body, conscious of any emotional areas.

**2.** Take seven deep, slow, and conscious breaths within a circle marked with candles, rope, rose petals, or fabric.

**3.** Gently touch your own chest and solar plexus to defuse any emotional areas.

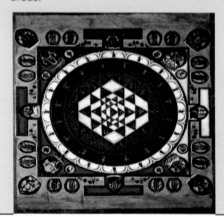

**4.** One of the two partners sits in front of the other and strokes the other's chest with a gentle and loving massage to awaken the feeling of containment. Then change roles.

**5.** Sitting in front, Shakti climbs on top of Shiva, hugging him gently. Do this slowly, feeling every movement.

**6.** In the circle that you made, meditate on the sounds you emit when inhaling and exhaling. Imagine that you are inside a circle of light.

**7.** Wait quietly, letting your souls merge, and feel the circle of energy that is formed between your bodies.

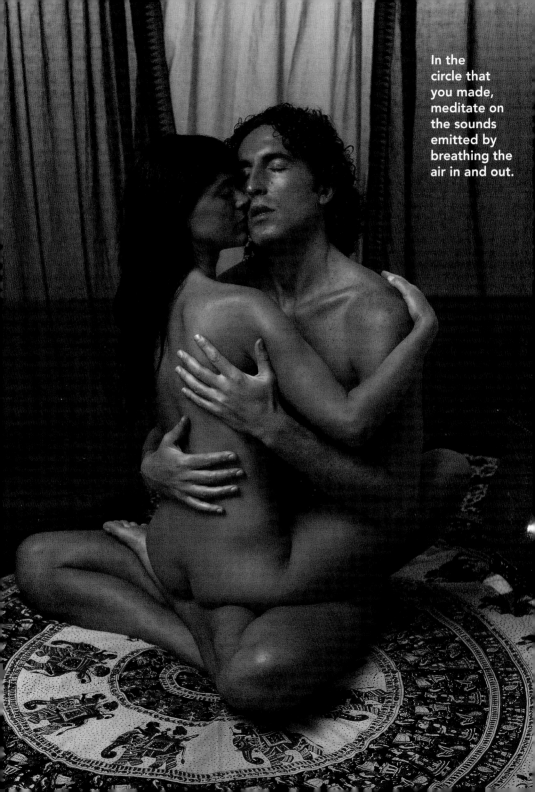

In the circle that you made, meditate on the sounds emitted by breathing the air in and out.

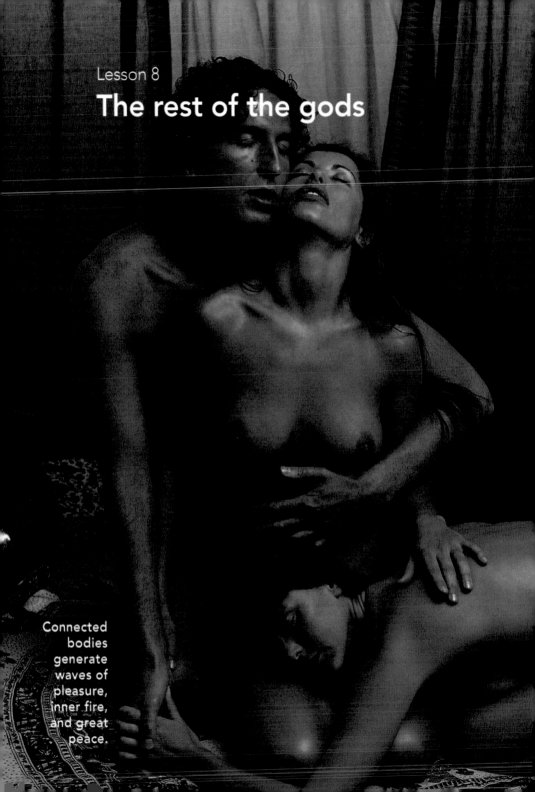

# The rest of the gods

Connected
bodies
generate
waves of
pleasure,
inner fire,
and great
peace.

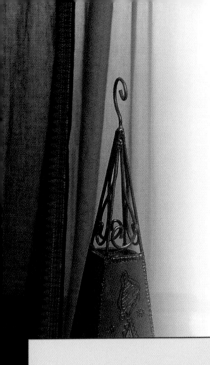

Wu Wei is known in the East, particularly in Japan, as the art of doing. We do things constantly, from thinking to action. This lesson teaches us to intoxicate our beings with no action and to delight in rest. It is said that after completing Creation, God rested on the seventh day—although from a Tantric perspective, I do not share this belief because Creation is constant and has never stopped.

**1.** On your bed or in a comfortable chair, lay naked, gently touching each other's bodies with your fingertips, or give each other massages with essential oils.

**2.** Do not speak, but let your mind let go of every thought while you slowly immerse yourself in silence.

**3.** Take deep breaths and exhale slowly by making the "Ahhhh" sound so that you can release tension with each exhalation.

**4.** Touch the entire body and erotic zones, including the genitals. Let electricity scroll across your body. Make love, as if in slow motion. Meditate together.

**5.** When you feel relaxed, lay together until you reach the state of Yoga Nidra, and "wash" your mind of worries and tension, taken over by complete rest.

In Tantra, there are two types of orgasms: from excitation and from relaxation.

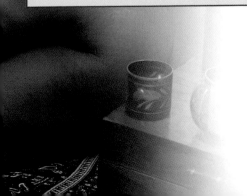

Lesson 9

# The science of breathing

In this ritual, you will share breath as the breath of life, as a vehicle of consciousness, as a connection that bridges energy and spirituality. Fe the flame of life.

**1.** Stand with your legs open, bring your arms to the floor, and inhale deeply. Then, go up the torso, undulating like a wave of energy, and lift your arms, exhaling loudly through the mouth, saying "Ahhhh." Repeat this several times, until you feel the movement as a wave of energy that is an action of the physical body.

**2.** Sitting face to face in the diamond position (with your legs bent or together) or with legs in a half lotus pose, get in touch through the third eye. Inhale through the nose while the other exhales and vice versa. Do this for at least fifteen minutes to half an hour: this will produce a powerful and deep energy exchange and will enrich the breath of life.

**3.** Lying hand in hand, begin to breathe in a circular method: inhale and exhale at a medium pace, four shallow breaths followed by one slow and deep breath. Do this cycle for ten minutes.

**4.** Stay relaxed through smooth, abdominal breathing, allowing energy to settle and harmonize, granting a state of peace. You can place your gems and quartz corresponding to each chakra during this final relaxation.

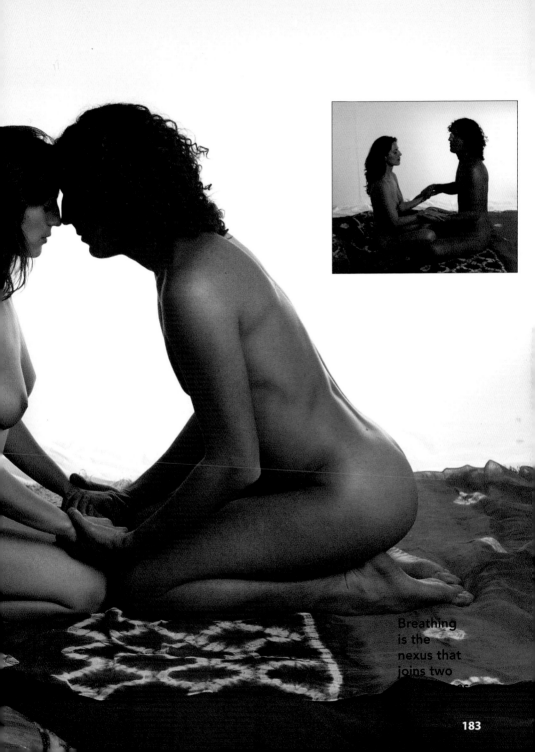

Breathing
is the
nexus that
joins two

# Sexual encounters during a full moon

The moon has a decisive influence on not only emotions, actions, and reactions, but also on sexual energy. The moon governs the tides, menstruation, plant growth, hair growth, etc.

We will harness the energy of the moon during its crescent phase during some of these lessons, and the full moon for this one in particular.

Tantra teaches Kundalini Shakti; "Every month, preferably during the full moon, assemble in one place in secret to worship me, as I am the queen of wisdom. You will then be freed from all bondage; as a symbol of freedom, you will be naked during these rites. Sing, rejoice, dance, play music, and make love, all in my presence, for I am both spiritual ecstasy and earthly enjoyment. My law is the love among all beings."

If possible, join one or more other couples to boost energy and benefit from the group—as we do in all of my courses—rise and multiply the effect of kundalini on your consciousness.

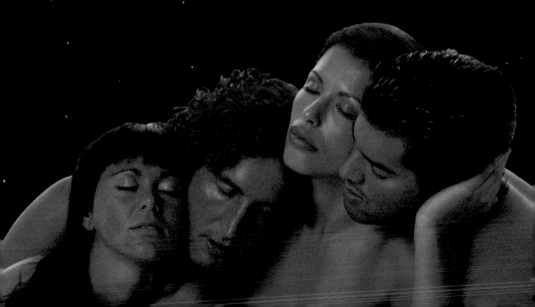

"Sing, rejoice, dance, play music, and make love, all in my presence."

**1.** Create a circle among the participants. Each will bring a white quartz in his hand. Meditate for fifteen minutes with the energy of the moon, visualizing how it enters the head, converts into saliva, and descends into the heart. Repeat the mantra *Om namah kundalini.*

**2.** Set the quartz at one side and join hands with each other to allow the energy of the circle to generate light.

**3.** Slide your hands to accentuate the sense of touch and generate electricity between bodies.

**4.** Once the energy has awakened, it will elevate you through a sensual dance, while blindfolded, so you can feel your world even deeper.

**5.** Shakti looks for Shiva with the palms of her hand until she makes contact with her dance partner. After a while, she dances with another Shakti.

**6.** Go back into the circle and meditate on the kundalini energy from the sacrum to the heart for several minutes. Let this work settle; this is the rising kundalini phase.

**7.** Recite the mantra seven times in honor of feminine energy and the moon.

**8.** Eat and drink in the presence of the vibrant energy of Shakti. If you can, perform this ritual with a view of the moon; meditate on it and then close your eyes to see through the third eye. Let the heart, body, and skin vibrate in joy and gladness.

## Lesson 11

# The wave and tantric scissors

These two sexual positions are important to contain ejaculation and extending the internal state as the wave of energy is mobilized to enter into meditation; the scissors can produce a slow and soft circuit of kundalini.

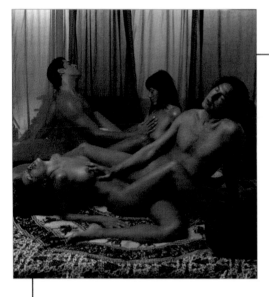

**2.** When you feel that you've had enough, stop the movement gradually until you are still with your backs straight.

**3.** Through the awakening of touch and the stimulation of conscious kisses, you can continue the erotic sensation.

**4.** When the climax of the internal fire ignites, stay for at least three conscious breaths. Shakti will open your yoni, the door of life, so that Shiva can enter the light wand, the lingam.

**1.** Shakti climbs on top of Shiva with her legs open and holds her heels behind his back. Begin to move forward and backward, breathing in unison so that you inhale as you move backward and exhale as you move forward. Breathing is a bridge, joining the movements and allowing entrance into a state of no mind.

**5.** With a slow and smooth penetration, move slowly, breathing in unison. Let pleasure extend throughout your body, from the genitals to the skin.

**6.** Intersperse the scissor position, with a wave of penetration. After a time, you will feel the connection that transcends the physical bodies.

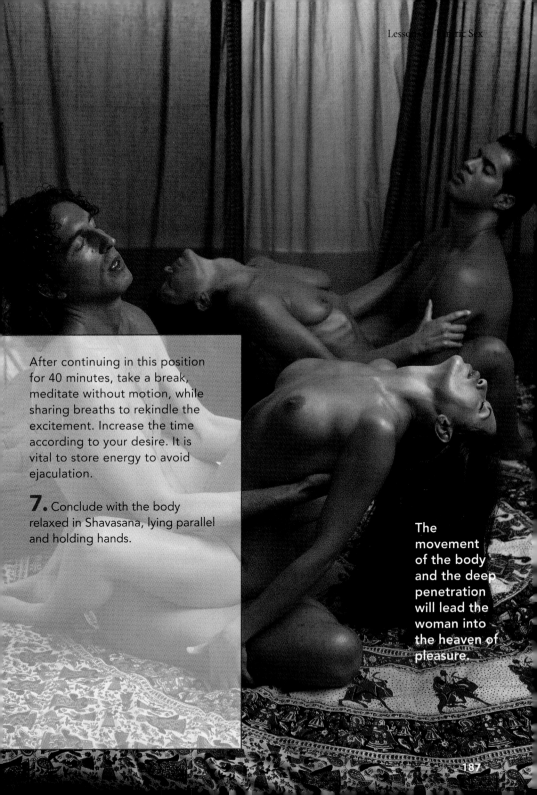

After continuing in this position for 40 minutes, take a break, meditate without motion, while sharing breaths to rekindle the excitement. Increase the time according to your desire. It is vital to store energy to avoid ejaculation.

**7.** Conclude with the body relaxed in Shavasana, lying parallel and holding hands.

The movement of the body and the deep penetration will lead the woman into the heaven of pleasure.

187

## Lesson 12

# Tantric meditation (active and passive)

Meditation is the art of harmonizing internal energy. We look at the silence of the mind as empowerment of kundalini energy. To do this, through Tantra, we practice dynamic meditation and also a more passive form.

The activity will make energy and power mobilize and harmonize the stillness, creating an internal state of joy and clarity.

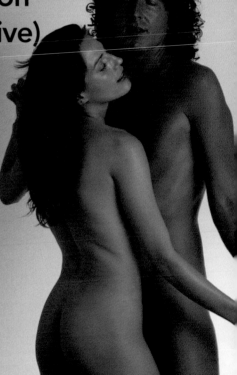

## 1. DYNAMIC TANTRIC MEDITATION

**First phase.** With rhythmic drum music, begin to unlock and mobilize the body for five minutes with cleansing breaths: inhale through the nose and exhale through the mouth.

**Second phase.** Continue with more dynamic drums or ethnic dance music, including percussion, for twenty minutes. The purpose of dancing is,

through deep breathing, to clean and energize the conscience and to become free. Moving the energy of consciousness will cause you to become more awake. Move all of the parts of the body: head, neck, shoulders, pelvis, legs, arms, etc.

**Third phase.** Lay on your back for ten minutes with soft music or in silence.

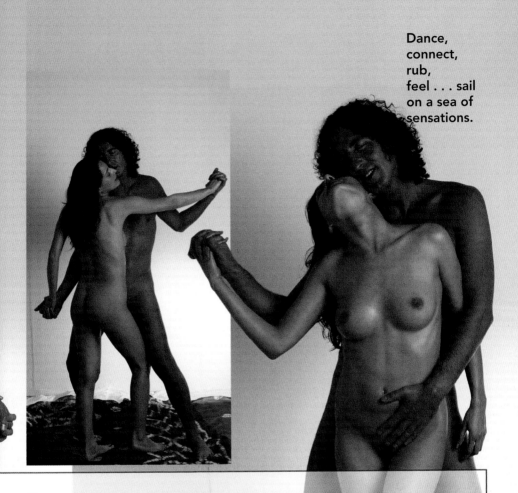

Dance,
connect,
rub,
feel . . . sail
on a sea of
sensations.

## 2. PASSIVE TANTRIC MEDITATION

**First phase.** In the Siddhasana or
Vajrasana position (lotus or diamond),
sit face to face. Breathe in unison for
five to ten minutes, holding hands to
improve energy flow between bodies.

**Second phase.** Focus all of the power
to the heart. Feel it rise from the first
chakra and feel all of the sexual energy
rise to anahatta, the chakra of love.

From there, visualize a loving stream of
pink and green light that feeds you.

**Third phase.** When you feel love
envelop you like a circle, let that energy
rise to the top of the head. This will be
the entrance to the top, the journey of
the human and animal and the human
and the divine.

Lesson 13

# The five elements and the five senses

Each element and each sense will take us five minutes; with the introduction of each new stimulus, continue to engage the previous sense and continue until all five are stimulated simultaneously.

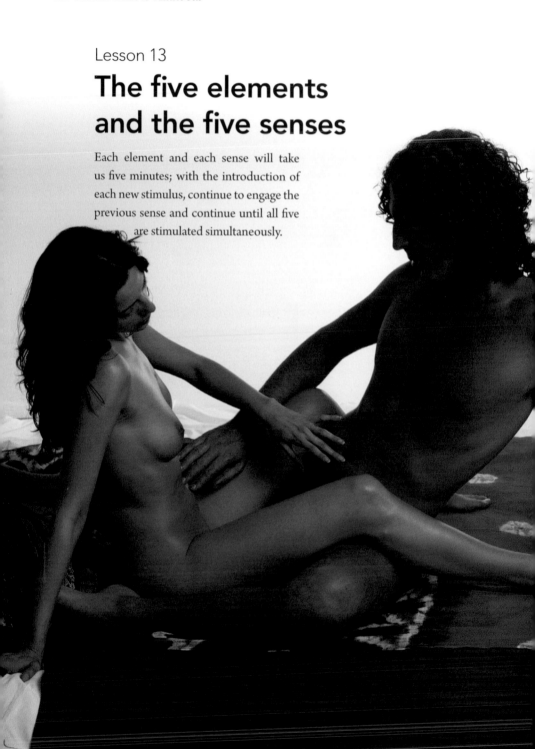

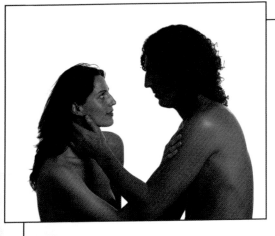

**7.** Visualize the water element as a river coming down from the mountain to join the deep sea. Imagine that you are bathing naked in calm, warm water. Place this meditation in the second chakra.

**8.** For fire, visualize a campfire in the countryside with flames, strength, and warmth. Place this meditation into the solar plexus, the third chakra.

**9.** Finally, the air element is located in the fourth chakra, in the center of the chest. You can view this as a flying eagle through the sky sharing your same journey.

**10.** Lying in silence, let the sum of the four elements enter into the cosmic ether, symbolizing the subtle and absolute.

**1.** Sitting opposite of each other, begin to touch each other with hands dipped in oil. Feel the hands of your partner and bring the energy of touch.

**2.** Continue looking deep into each other's eyes.

**3.** Close your eyes and devote five minutes to the power of hearing, listening to each other's breathing.

**4.** Follow by stimulating the sense of smell, taking in the distinct odor of the other.

**5.** Finally, stimulate the sense of taste with soft kisses.

**6.** Stay motionless to enter into the meditation of the elements. Start to visualize the earth element as a meadow, a valley, or a field of corn. Place this meditation in the first chakra.

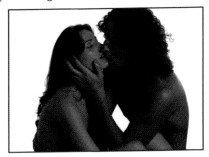

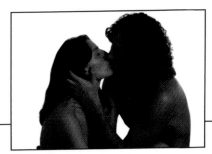

Lesson 14

# How to enter the tantric orgasm

In Tantra, orgasm can be compared to the great cosmic explosion, the *Big Bang*—a powerful state in which the divine manifests in the human body. Most women do not get to experience a real orgasm during their lives and men believe that ejaculation is the culmination of the sexual act. With tantric techniques you can find states that are latent, hidden, and repressed. Orgasm is a natural ability, and by natural I mean a gift from God, intrinsic to human nature. The word "orgasm" has to do with "agency" and "orgy" and "organization." Orgasm is the door leading to the divinity in every human being.

**Begin to awaken the erotic points around the body.**

Valerie Brooks says in her boo[k] *Tantra Para Mujeres* (*Tantra f[or] Women*), "when my heart finall[y] allowed me to venture inside, [a] thousand words could not describ[e] what I saw. Within this vast cent[er] is not the essence, the substanc[e] of the heart: there is much mor[e.] Here lies the whole universe, ever[y]thing, everything that I see outsid[e] myself, plus all of the other plan[es] of existence. It is everything. It [is] the residence of the gods: Moth[er] and Father. Therefore, this path [of] liberation begins and continues [at] the ends of the heart.

I felt a wave of joy and returne[d] to fall into a slow rhythmic embra[ce] of my lover. I felt in the center of t[he] heart a sexual energy deposited [in] this soft, sweet, and infinite spac[e.] When I reached orgasm, I felt a[n] explosion, as if a star had expl[oded] so big that I could[n't] thin[k of any]thing, I couldn['t] [se]e [and I] saw a glimpse of [a] [whit]e light. My body con[vul]s[ed,] my [mind] was blank. Yes, [we are] all mad[e of] stardust."

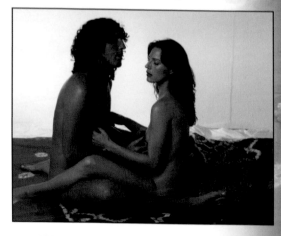

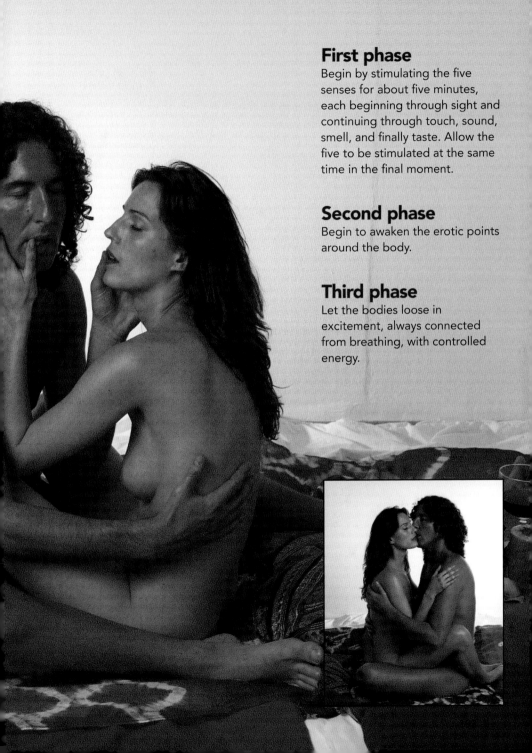

### First phase

Begin by stimulating the five senses for about five minutes, each beginning through sight and continuing through touch, sound, smell, and finally taste. Allow the five to be stimulated at the same time in the final moment.

### Second phase

Begin to awaken the erotic points around the body.

### Third phase

Let the bodies loose in excitement, always connected from breathing, with controlled energy.

## Fourth phase

Stimulate the lingam and yoni with oral sex; this can happen simultaneously in the 69 position.

## Fifth phase

Begin penetration in the Yab-Yum position with a slow pace until reaching a crescendo before stopping. Then, meditate in stillness and breathe in unison, which turns into energy. Build this up and then stop; do this at least three times. Orgasmic energy is latent power.

## Sixth phase

Let the power of the female orgasm rise. It is important to stimulate the anus with Shiva's middle finger in order to feel Shakti's orgasmic contractions.

By feeling these contractions, you know that the orgasm is rea

## Seventh phase

Stimulate Shiva in the center of his chest, his fourth chakra, especially his nipples in order to wake the other poles of energy. Visualizing and breathing bring energy to the heart and then the rest of the body. You will feel the flow of electricity throughout the body through convulsions and arching, modeled after the vibrant energy of orgasm withou ejaculation, but he will return to normal after a few minutes. This orgasm is global, decentralizing only the genital area but involving the entire body. Finish with the "X" position, relaxing.

> Stimulate the lingam and yoni with oral sex; this can happen simultaneously in the 69 position.

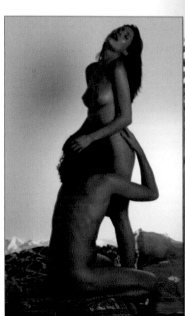

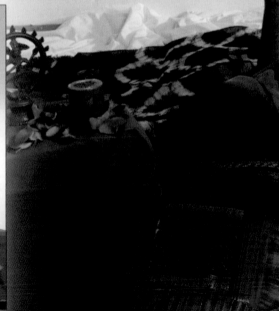

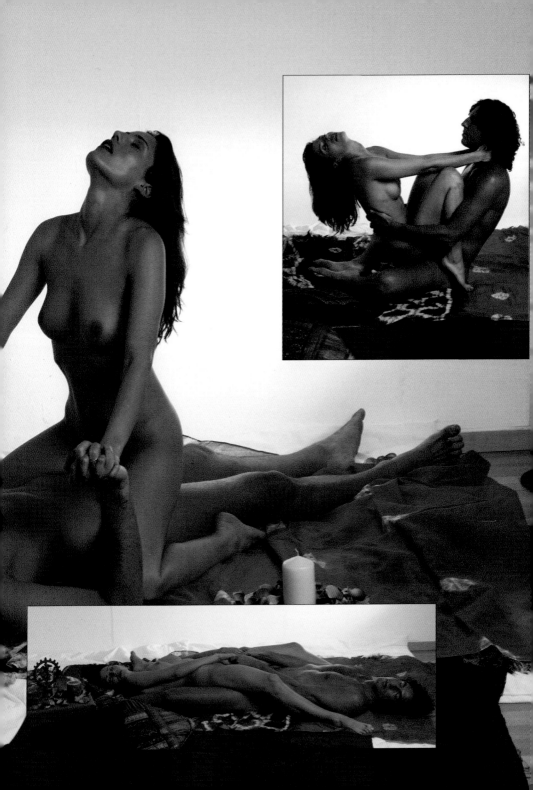

Lesson 15

# The sexual ritual "maithuna"

The *maithuna* is a sexual ritual between Shiva and Shakti to not only enhance the orgasmic state, but also the spiritual fusion. In the encounter between the woman and the man, in their nudity and vibrant bodies, their excitement, meditative ability, eroticism and sensuality, and the liberation of the senses, the supreme joy is celebrated. The *maithuna* is a ritual of *sadhana*, the tantric workout.

In the East, sex is "prescribed" as a medicine against disease, depression, and anxiety. For Tantra, this is the supreme knowledge of the fusion of the divine energized through physical bodies.

**Important:** Tantric couples will have an intention beforehand. They will coordinate what they want to enhance in the ritual in order to focus the energy. It is not advis-

able to enter this ritual without a specific intention, as the energy will be dispersed and lost. The tantric know that where thinking goes, energy goes.

**Coat the body with oils or perfumes and stimulate with musk, sandalwood, jasmine, or larosa oil incense.**

## First phase

Take a refreshing and purifying bath. Coat the body with oils or perfumes and stimulate with musk, sandalwood, jasmine, or larosa oil incense.

## Second phase

Stretch the naked body through yoga poses.

## Third phase

Dance soft and meditative dances to candlelight.

## Fourth phase

Provide mutual massages to relax from stresses and to enhance the sense of touch.

## Fifth phase

Share food (cereal, meat, fish, or wine) and open up to sex. Exercise polarized breathing (solar-lunar), alternating breaths through each nostril. Complete seven complete cycles (see my other book, *The Art of Tantra*, from the same publisher).

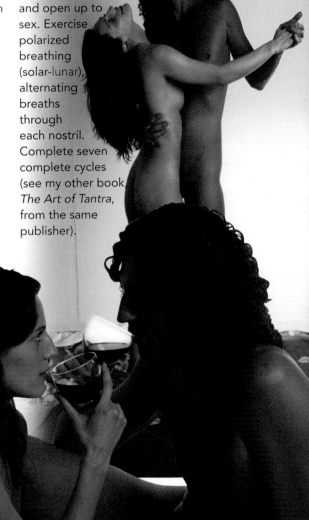

## Sixth phase

Once your breathing is connected, do it through both nostrils at the same time while chanting the mantra OM or *OmÁ bhurÁbwaÁswaja.*

## Seventh phase

Perform an act to honor Shiva and Shakti by offering a prayer, a candle, some flowers, or even candy. This also serves to remind the unconscious self of the sacredness of the ritual.

## Eighth phase

For a few minutes, visualize the flame of a candle, feeling the light in each heart. Then close your eyes and focus on the third eye, the ajna chakra, which is the point of command of all chakras.

## Ninth phase

While meditating on the system of chakras, visualize them as colorful flowers that open and enlarge.

## Tenth phase

In the yab-yum posture, stimulate each other with your hands and mouth. Shiva will ask permission to enter the yoni of Shakti, the gate of life. Shakti accepts and opens her lips and Shiva will be sweet, smooth, and strong at the same time in order to feel with deep sensibility the impact of their union.

In the yab-yum posture, stimulate each other with your hands and mouth. Shiva will ask permission to enter the yoni of Shakti.

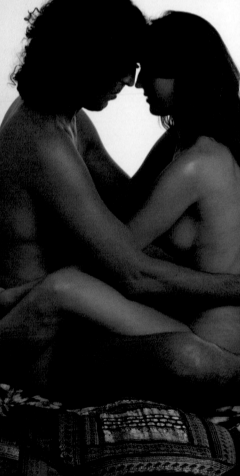

## Eleventh phase

With very few movements, meditate and feel your sexual energy at the same time. Sex and meditation in a circle of light that joins the cosmic couple. You can extend this game for hours. If orgasm is reached, then you must focus on prior intention, opening the inner eye so that inner light can spread. This sexual magic is powerful, and if all the energy that has been awoken between both parties is directed to each other, there is a better chance for that power to be concrete.

## Twelfth phase

Relax; share food and wine. You can stay in meditation or dance in celebration.

Osho says, "Tantra is focused on another type of orgasm. If we call the first class the 'peak orgasm,' you can call the tantric orgasm the 'valley orgasm.' This is because you are not reaching the peak of excitement, but the deepest valley of relaxation. The excitation comes from the couple at the beginning. This is why, in the beginning, orgasms are equal, but in the end, they are different. For the first, the excitement has to be

intense . . . more and more intense. You have to grow into it, you have to help it grow towards its peak.

Then excitement is just the beginning. And once the man has entered, both the lover and beloved, they can relax. No movement is required. They can relax in a loving embrace.

When a man or woman begins to feel that he is losing his erection, they only have to move a little bit to feel relaxed again.

You can prolong this deep embrace for hours without ejaculation, and then you can come together into a deep sleep. This is the valley orgasm. You are relaxed, and you find yourself relaxed as two beings. The ordinary sexual orgasm looks crazy. The tantric orgasm is a relaxed and profound meditation. You can be gratified all you want because you will not lose any energy, but it will increase. By simply meeting with the opposite pole, your energy will be renewed. The act of tantric love can be done as many times as you want. Basic sex cannot because you lose energy and your body has to wait, only to lose energy again."

**You can prolong this deep embrace for hours without ejaculation, then later you can enter her.**

## Lesson 16

# Tantra for women

Every woman is a delight for the eyes, the hands, and the mystery of life. Every woman is a beautiful goddess, a piece of heaven on earth. We are born by women, we leave through her!

My vision as a tantric, plus as a man, is that woman is poetry for the soul. I do not say this as a prudish cliche. Every Shiva without a Shakti is a Shava, a corpse. The woman is the impulse, the muse, the instinct of life, the mystery of nature, the ability to show harmony at work, to see your body and actions. Women do not incite war—only gossip from television programs.

The woman is the engine, terrain, fertile field where we sow the seeds of life—not only for new children, but for every single day. I have personally delighted in the divine benefits of the women I've met, but the tantric companion who has given me the universe is beautiful, smart, and multiorgasmic, and I was able to seduce her several years ago with chocolate and a violet-scented letter. While the tantric way implies abundance, comfort, and enjoyment (though not posessive), her

**Dance to a softer, more sensual, slower, and more meditative pace. Feel that you are a goddess and dance to your beloved or alone with the entire universe.**

**1.** With the naked body, dance to the sound of drums and wild rhythmic music.

**2.** Breathe, panting like an animal in heat. Let your instincts awaken without barriers: scream, jump, enjo liberate.

**3.** Now dance to a softer, more sensual, slower, and more meditativ pace. Feel that you are a goddess and dance to your beloved or alone with the entire universe.

**4.** Spread aromatic oils all over your body and awaken the sexual energy in all of your erotic points.

**5.** Connect with the feminine energy. Imagine that you are a flow and that the orgasmic perfume of your life spreads everywhere.

stay impacted that. I realized that the woman is entered through the heart and not the vagina. This is a part of the tantric history of lights, valleys, and mountains where there emerge the clear waters of understanding and learning. Through this, I learned many, many lessons.

**6.** Stimulate the crown jewel: the clitoris, nipples, and the G-spot. Many women do not know where this is. To discover it, enter the upper wall of the yoni, about five or eight centimeters, with your finger. This is a point that produces pleasurable stimuli in the brain.

**7.** Breathe in the sexual energy and put it into every pore of your skin. Remember that you are the one who dominates the energy.

**8.** Relax and bring your hands to your chest, leaving the heart relaxed; the body is vibrant and awake, the soul is free.

Lesson 17

# Secret sexual initiations and games

**Children innocently touch their own bodies and they are pure.**

**Tantra is a road to power through the unity of Shiva and Shakti** as a cosmic couple, but that does not preclude participants having more meditative sex with a sacred consciousness.

Several spiritual, sexual initiations take place through a tantric partner, a woman or a man. While it may seem like a bad religious practice (sexuality variants are the order of the day throughout the world), the tantric ritual is performed to pool conscious energy and to wake archetypes of the unconscious. For example, if you eat meat and could choose, how would you prefer the animals

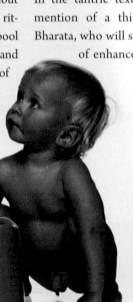

you eat be sacrificed: in a brutal way (as is done habitually) or as a sacred ritual offering to the divine? For ordinary sex acts, without ritual, without more than the attraction, are ordinary, while Tantra is performed on special occasions as a way to worship the divine.

In the Christian Trinity, there is the Father, Son, and Holy Spirit: there is no female divinity. In Tantra, there is a matriarchal road; it looks for the most feminine energy. In the tantric texts, there is the mention of a third companion, Bharata, who will share the secrets of enhanced energy.

Children touch their genitals naturally. They are investigating and exploring new feelings. Adults then start to admonish them: "Don't touch that," or "don't do that," or "yuck," etc. This is the first sexual trauma. Touching is synonymous with feeling, knowing, and pleasure. Why do we condemn pleasure? Tantra is pure, innocent, and natural. Attraction, feeling, unity, meditation, ecstasy...all for a natural environment! Life has given us sex in order to feel divine! Let innocence return to your mind and especially to your body. Religion has mutilated sex; now it's time for purification, and Tantra is the art that makes the soul shine through the extended use of sexual energy attached to meditation.

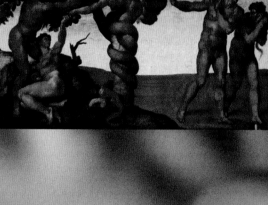

Original sin is a repressed, condemnatory seed. Tantra brings freedom.

# Tantric ritual of the trinity

**1.** Take three participants, naked and holding hands while forming a triangle with their bodies.

**2.** Forgetting the impulses of the personality of possession or jealousy, you will feel that Shakti is in each woman and that Shiva is in each man. You have to repeat the mantra *Om Shakti hum* and afterward *Om namah shivaia* and then focus your energies on Shiva.

**3.** Begin to stimulate the senses, touching the bodies with aromatic oils. Let the sexual fire grow and distribute it in order to breathe.

**4.** Then you will allow all of the senses to be stimulated: smelling, kissing, and listening to the sounds of love.

**5.** One of the Shaktis will be stimulated with caresses and other forms of pleasure by the other two. Then after bringing her to ecstasy, the other companion will also be stimulated. Finally, Shiva will receive their essence of yin. You share bodies, kissing and cuddling until the fire is raised high.

**6.** Shakti receives the lingam of Shiva and Shakti invites the caress and meditates in the act of love. Shakti will repeat "I receive and accept you."

Then, when satisfied, Shiva will be invited to penetrate the same way. At all times, energy is shared through breathing and consciousness through the divine act without degrading the act like that of an animal; pure sexual awareness will remain. We must seize to power and charge your chakras with this powerful stream of fire that was generated.

**7.** After hours have passed and the three parts of the Trinity are satisfied and full, through fun games, let your bodies settle on the most exquisite relaxations while meditating on the energy of sexual attraction and the power of the triangle shape. You will eat tasty dishes, you will dance and taste good wine, and you will immerse in Yoga Nidra, a meditative break from the gods.

**Note:** The man will have an orgasm like Shakti, but he will not lose his bindu, i.e., will not ejaculate, without using all of the yin energy received to enhance his inner woman, creativity, sensuality, and spiritual connection. This is an advanced practice fas much or women as it is also a litmus test for the man.

Let the waves of bliss and pleasure extend and hold; bear in mind at all times that any vertex of the triangle cannot be more important than the others. The key to success of the ritual is balance.

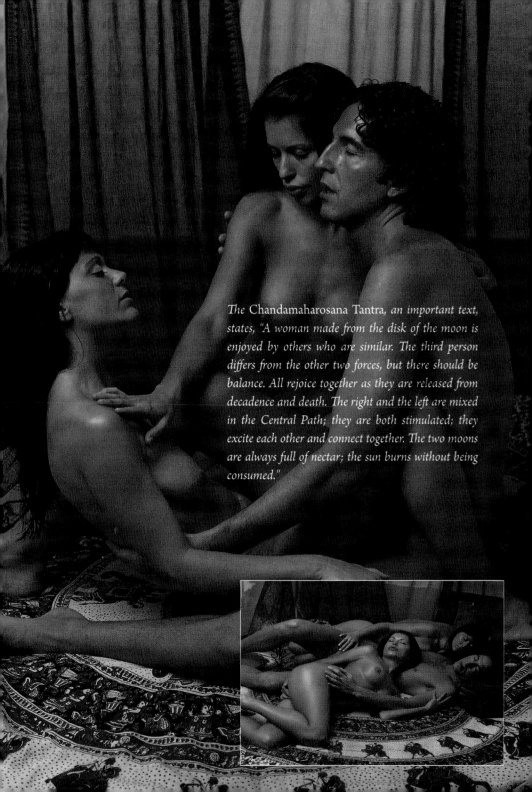

The Chandamaharosana Tantra, an important text, states, "A woman made from the disk of the moon is enjoyed by others who are similar. The third person differs from the other two forces, but there should be balance. All rejoice together as they are released from decadence and death. The right and the left are mixed in the Central Path; they are both stimulated; they excite each other and connect together. The two moons are always full of nectar; the sun burns without being consumed."

Lesson 18

# Tantra for groups

Among the sexual initiations of Tantra, this is the *Chakra puja*, which means "wheel of ecstasy" or "circular cult." This ritual is performed between eight couples, but can also be made with four participants (two tantric couples) if there exists the sacred consciousness.

In ancient times, many cultures performed sexual rituals in nature to ensure a good harvest and fertility. In Greece, for example, the term "orgy" appeared in the rituals dedicated to the god Dionysus.

While in the West, most people are frightened at the idea. These rituals date back to the dawn of time. The naturalness of sex was such that no problems, taboos, or conditions, existed. Religion has poisoned sex without killing it; it is half dead, maimed. Tantra is a "medicine" (a word whose root is "meditate") that heals sexual wounds. While this ritual is advanced and requires a lot of patience, I cannot fail to mention it here.

The psychologist Wilhelm Reich thoroughly investigated the power of sexual energy, and what

Tantra looks for with this ritual (not required) is the lighting of individual consciousness through the collective consciousness.

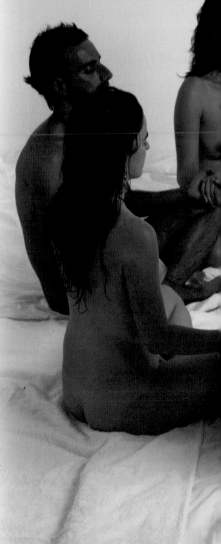

**All of the participants are nude in a circle, with a fire burning in the center, and the group guru leads the exercise.**

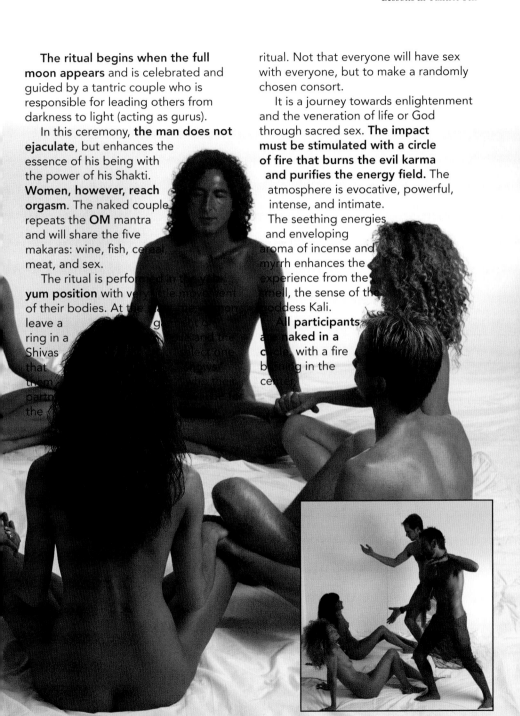

The ritual begins when the full moon appears and is celebrated and guided by a tantric couple who is responsible for leading others from darkness to light (acting as gurus).

In this ceremony, the man does not ejaculate, but enhances the essence of his being with the power of his Shakti. Women, however, reach orgasm. The naked couple repeats the OM mantra and will share the five makaras: wine, fish, cereal, meat, and sex.

The ritual is performed in the yab-yum position with very little movement of their bodies. At the same time, men leave a ... ring in a ... Shivas ... that ... them ... part ... the ...

ritual. Not that everyone will have sex with everyone, but to make a randomly chosen consort.

It is a journey towards enlightenment and the veneration of life or God through sacred sex. The impact must be stimulated with a circle of fire that burns the evil karma and purifies the energy field. The atmosphere is evocative, powerful, intense, and intimate. The seething energies and enveloping aroma of incense and myrrh enhances the experience from the smell, the sense of the goddess Kali.

All participants are naked in a circle with a fire burning in the center.

and the group guru leads the exercise. After repeating the mantras and sharing makaras, **the Shaktis offer their dance as a gift of life, an example of sensuality, beauty, and power. The Shivas will then do the same for them.** Dancing is a symbol of cosmic motion, as the supreme eternal dancers. **Pursue a sensual massage among all of the participants** with their eyes closed until the sexual current invades the skin. Touch will be the vehicle that connects the group; touch and be touched without resistance, subtly with fire. Next couples are placed back to back to enhance the energy of the chakras and begin to mobilize slowly, gently rubbing their spines, which will generate even more heat. **The passion vibrates**

**and stimulates sexual energy between partners until the instructor gives the signal for the consummation of the bodies.** Beforehand, take deep breaths in order to channel sexual energy to the heart.

Upon penetrating Shakti, Shiva enters in the mysteries of life. To be penetrated, Shakti leaves her metaphysical and magical feminine scent free and sensitive to the environment. Energies rise and controlled passion is channeled into the above column for all of the chakras; conscious breathing, subtle body movements, the prolongation for hours . . . everything boils, life throbs, and the atmosphere is pure light . . . .

The moans, voices, rhythms, and breathing are the language with which Tantra speaks to life in this magical night. **Several hours later, the ritual ends with the repetition of mantras and deep meditation in search of inner light.** When energy is harmonized, the night is an invitation to Yoga Nidra. Everyone sleeps intertwined together. Many tantric initiations occur in the astral plane, in the hours of sleep. The energy that has remained in the room powers auras, chakras, and the psyche all participants.

The ancestral ritual of reverence of life, the essence of divinity of each one, has been celebrated; the sun shines in your eyes and the fire in your hearts and smile on your faces show happiness and shared joy. In short, the raw materials from which life is made: pure delight.

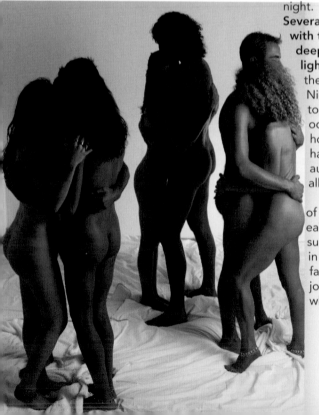

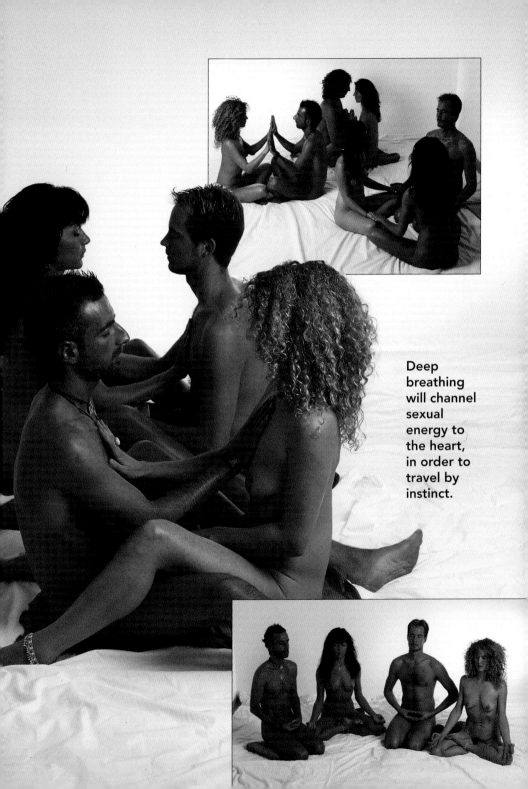

Deep
breathing
will channel
sexual
energy to
the heart,
in order to
travel by
instinct.

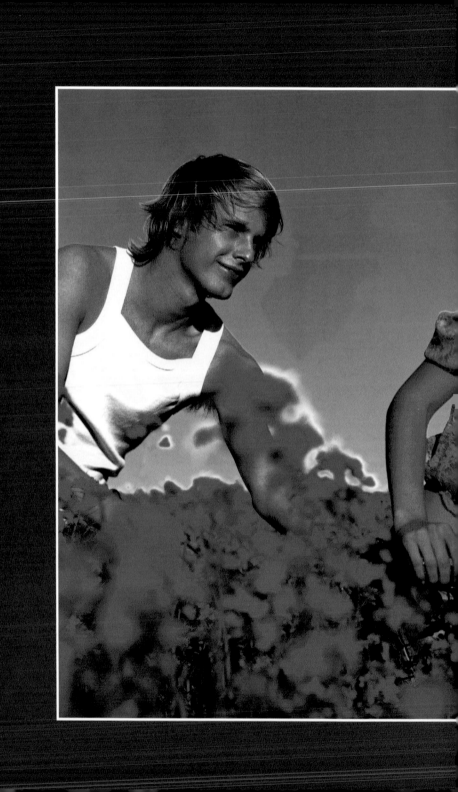

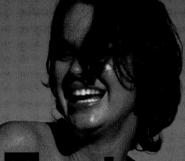

# Tantra in your daily life

*"Listen to your heart, feel it live, at the explosive time and in peace. Live every moment entirely."*

GUILLERMO FERRARA

# Be true to yourself

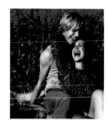

Fidelity is hearing the heart; if you are true to yourself, your soul, to the deep zone of your being, you'll never be unfaithful with your partner or friends. **"Infidelity"** means listening to the voice of selfishness, which seeks to conquer or possess another body.

Usually we refer to infidelity when it comes to sexual encounters with other people who are not your partner. The male wants to penetrate a new female and the woman feels free with another man. Keep in mind that there is the desire, the attraction between opposites, but my suggestion (if you have opened a door, it will only allow you to realize that the circle of illusory experiences leads inevitably to valuing the real person you love) is that you cultivate your link with the momentum and zeal of an artist who is creating a work of genius. It is good to remember that there is no greater miracle than to find your other half and share your life with her.

The relation of the tantric couple is **artistic**, because they become *artists* in love.

Discover the details that make life great with a partner: create, surprise, excite, motivate, change, learn, enjoy, celebrate, travel, love, feel, give, serve, innovate.... There are so many things to ensure that the fire of love stays lit! In this way there will be no need to seek something external. It may be that we let ourselves be consumed by routine or "taken for granted" the other, and only when the value is gone. For this not to happen, we must cultivate intimacy, which is something supreme and unique.

It is worth learning that when you have a sacred bond, you should protect it like you would a flower in a storm. Until you find this connection, experiment with various people, but when the heart tells you that this is the person you want to be in the universe, do not hesitate for a moment. Listen to it!

> **There is no greater miracle than finding your other half and sharing your life with her.**

## 10 tantric suggestions

The word "command" denotes some[one who] obeys the commands of another. I pre[fer] to give some personal suggestions ba[sed] on my experience (I don't say advice because the ignorant are not going to follow and the wise do not need it).

1. Tell your lover if it is real love.
2. Live entirely without divisions.
3. Evaluate your interior and your privacy.
4. Share life with your partner in a creative and sacred way.
5. Accept the world as a divine school.
6. Live from the heart and intelligence.
7. Be true to yourself.
8. Expand your consciousness every day.
9. Celebrate each moment.
10. Impose these upon yourself, based on your own personal wisdom.

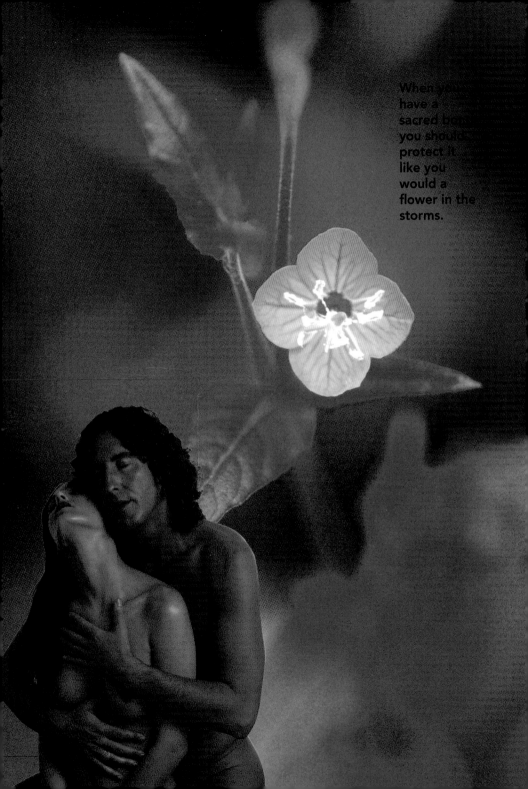

When you
have a
sacred body
you should
protect it
like you
would a
flower in the
storms.

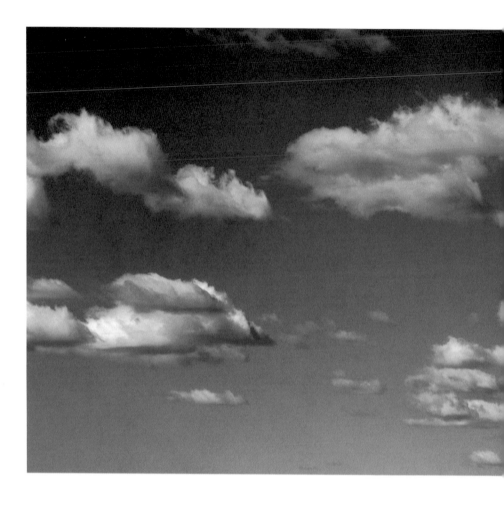

Heaven is in
your heart.

# From Earth to
# Heaven in a breath

We have been taught to think erroneously that heaven, paradise, is something external. There is no more paradise or hell than there is within ourselves. A personal paradise must be built; for example, through positive attitudes, with love, with creative thoughts, through conscious living of the present and cultivating fun and loving personal relationships, by valuing the person you love, by taking care of yourself . . . .

Living well does not require much money, but rather creativity. No need to keep working at home from the office; don't overload yourself

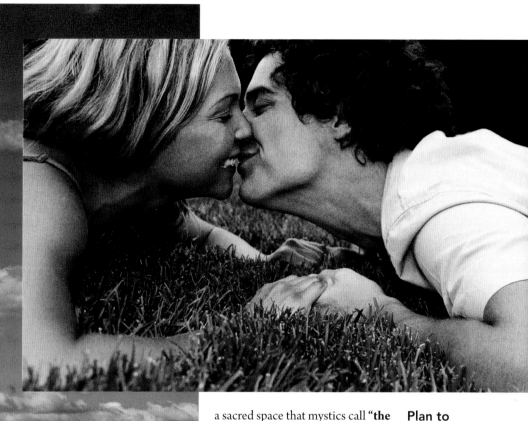

a sacred space that mystics call **"the inner sky,"** the self, the soul.

Feeling that you can connect to that voice is one of the first steps in your day-to-day heaven. Tantra connects (one cannot separate, even if he wants to) the material the earthly, and the mundane with the divine; the spiritual and emotional aspirations. One should be trained to combine work and relaxation, meditation and money, the earthly and the spiritual, because they are all woven by the same hand.

with problems or let being tired keep you from making love, meditating, giving or receiving a good massage, preparing a good menu, practicing yoga, or laughing with friends.

There are several ways to get to know yourself inside; one of them is meditation. You can breathe deeply and gradually go beyond the limits of the rational mind; you will enter

**Plan to train yourself to combine the earthly and the spiritual because they are woven by the same hand.**

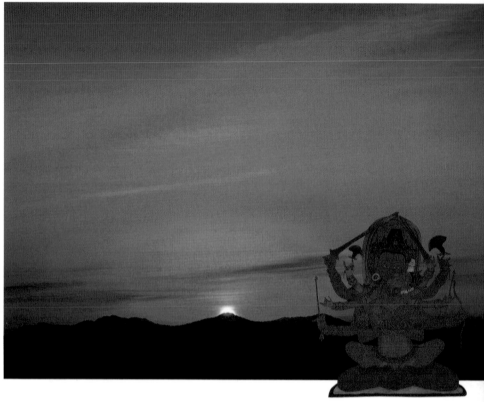

## Emotions: keys to the inner self

**Take advantage of the energy of the crescent and full moon, as they are important in daily tantric life.**

The tantric path consists, among other things, of obtaining the expertise of emotions. Clearly there are times when certain emotions disrupt your vision and we react through our impulses and hormones rather than responding through awareness and maturity.

Therefore, we must master holding back anger, worry, sadness, and loneliness, and focus our energy on adventure, excitement, trust, lovingness, compassion, creativity, and hope. Positive emotions spin the wheel of our lives, the wheel of the chakras and psyche, into bright, personal happiness. But remember, light becomes most important when it passes through the darkness. Paul, before he became a saint, was a persecutor of the divine, a dark being, until something changed him inside when he realized what is divine.

Light is much more intense when it emerges from the darkness, as it simply disappears with the luminosity of positive emotions as we direct our being from pleasure to consciousness.

## The moon and Tantra

Harnessing the power of the crescent and full moon is important in daily tantric life in order to perform rituals, to raise kundalini energy, and to harmonize the emotions.

It is known, in these two phases of the moon, that there is more energy reflected from the sun and that this greatly influences human beings. There must be a prevention of ejaculation, for example, because if this sexual energy is not channeled through a creative and loving end, it is likely that the full moon will affect us negatively (with anger, for example).

Right now we should apply the techniques that allow us to specify the intention to grow any facet of our lives; in this way we will make this energy flow and not cause harm. The moon is a female element and an ally in the tantric way. In the next two phases, i.e., when it is waning and dark, it is convenient to practice in order to maintain energy.

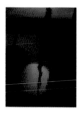

**A time of loneliness is a time of light, of inner sun.**

## Don't listen to your brain

*"Today I am rich: I have no memory."*
JAUME SISA

The mind can be a real impediment to Tantra; considering that it is so useful and necessary for certain things, it is a real nuisance in the field of meditation and personal transformation.

The mind can censor emotions and feelings, so you run the risk of being dissatisfied and repressed. The rigid and repressive ideas of the mind can block the body. Nakedness, for example, can be seen by the mind as something abnormal or weird. The mind speculates; the heart delivers.

Do not forget that the tantric road begins with the body and the heart, bypassing the mind.

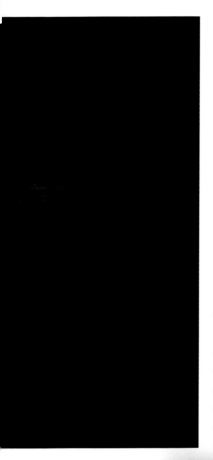

do not see it during the moment of teaching, we do much later.

## Tantric solitude

There are times when being alone is necessary in order to drink from the internal fountain. Loneliness can hurt and not be constructive, but it is also a way to learn so that when we find someone who we love, we can fill ourselves with devotion.

The first step is to love ourselves—in a good way—we are the same, and the time of loneliness is a time of light, an internal sun. We have to pass this difficult ordeal of accepting that we are alone even though we are surrounded by people. This loneliness allows us to discover the divine within ourselves. When the fire ignites, the entire universe is with you and guides you towards the realization of your destiny.

Tantra, remember, is a path to return to innocence, wisdom, delivery, and trust, and all pass through the open heart and not through padlocks of the mind.

When mental fears (often illusory) arise, put your hand on your chest, breathe deeply, and trust. The divine is always there to help; although we

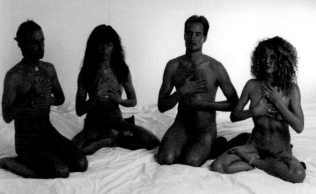

# How to creatively use sexual energy: the 64 arts

While the *Sa ́ a ̄t d æ*("kama": "desire"; "sutra": "wisdom") does not belong to the tantric encyclopedia, as it came later, this agreement was written in Sanskrit by the hand of Vastyayana, a sage in India, and is greatly useful in understanding what to do with sexual energy and how we can funnel it into an art form.

Kama, the god of love (the Hindu version of Cupid), is the path for obtaining spiritual transcendence. Kama can also be understood as the cosmic desire, the creative impulse.

Both women and men know that tantrics have to master these arts to find their embodiments. A person may feel tantric when she masters the 64 arts, including the art of sex. Many people mistakenly say, "I am tantric," because they are able to make love for a few hours without ejaculating. Tantra is much more than that; it is a special inner attitude: mystical, pragmatic, sexual, scientific, artistic, and celebratory.

> The *Kama Sutra* mentions the need to harmonize the three qualities of life:
>
> **1.** The spiritual merit (Dharma)
> **2.** Economic prosperity (Artha)
> **3.** Sexual satisfaction (Kama)

In ancient India, before marriage, women were instructed in the arts of life. A tantric teacher who masters these arts becomes a powerful, creative, intelligent, and loving being with great value. Therefore, it is important to know that after triggering sparks of sex and the internal birth of the loving state, you can release a huge wave of fullness and creativity in the following activities:

1. Singing
2. Playing on musical instruments
3. Dancing
4. Union of dancing, singing, and playing instrumental music
5. Writing and drawing
6. Tattooing
7. Arraying and adorning an idol with rice and flowers
8. Spreading and arranging beds or couches of flowers, or flowers upon the ground
9. Coloring the teeth, garments, hair, nails and bodies, i.e. staining, dyeing coloring and painting the same
10. Fixing stained glass into a floor
11. The art of making beds, and spreading out carpets and cushions for reclining
12. Playing on musical glasses filled with water
13. Storing and accumulating water in aqueducts, cisterns, and reservoirs
14. Picture making, trimming and decorating
15. Stringing of rosaries, necklaces, garlands and wreaths
16. Binding of turbans and chaplets, and making crests and top-knots of flowers

17. Scenic representations, stage playing
18. The art of making ear ornaments
19. The art of preparing perfumes and odors
20. Proper disposition of jewels and decorations, and adornment in dress
21. Magic or sorcery
22. Quickness of hand or manual skill
23. Culinary art, i.e. cooking and cookery
24. Making drinks with or without alcohol
25. Tailor's work and sewing
26. Making parrots, flowers, tufts, tassels, bunches, bosses, knobs, etc., out of yarn or thread
27. Solution of riddles, enigmas, covert speeches, verbal puzzles, and enigmatical questions
28. Games with verses
29. The art of mimicry or imitation
30. Reading, including chanting and intoning
31. Study of sentences difficult to pronounce. It is played as a game chiefly by women and children
32. Practice with sword, single stick, quarter staff, and bow and arrow
33. Drawing inferences, reasoning, or inferring
34. Carpentry, or the work of a carpenter
35. Architecture, or the art of building
36. Knowledge about gold and silver coins, and jewels and gems
37. Chemistry and mineralogy
38. Coloring jewels, gems, and beads
39. Knowledge of mines and quarries
40. Cultivating, taking care of, and growing plants
41. The art of cock fighting, quail fighting and ram fighting
42. The art of teaching parrots and starlings to speak
43. The art of applying perfumed ointments to the body, and of dressing the hair with unguents and perfumes and braiding it
44. The art of understanding writing in cipher, and the writing of words in a peculiar way
45. The art of speaking by changing the forms of words
46. Knowledge of language and of the vernacular dialects
47. The art of making flower carriages
48. The art of framing mystical diagrams, of addressing spells and charms, and binding armlets
49. Mental exercises, such as completing stanzas or verses
50. Composing poems
51. Knowledge of dictionaries and vocabularies
52. Knowledge of ways of changing and disguising the appearance of persons
53. Knowledge of the art of changing the appearance of things
54. Various ways of gambling
55. The art of obtaining possession of the property of others by means of mantras or incantations
56. Skill in youthful sports
57. Behaving in society
58. Knowledge of the art of war
59. Knowledge of gymnastics
60. The art of knowing the character of a man from his features
61. Knowledge of scanning or constructing verses
62. Arithmetical recreations
63. Making artificial flowers
64. Making figures and images in clay

When a person masters and has knowledge of these arts, he increases his value; he will be honored wherever he goes. With these arts, says the *Kama Sutra*, anyone could easily win at life even while living in a foreign country. Knowledge is very attractive and Tantra ensures immediate success with both women and men.

Practice!

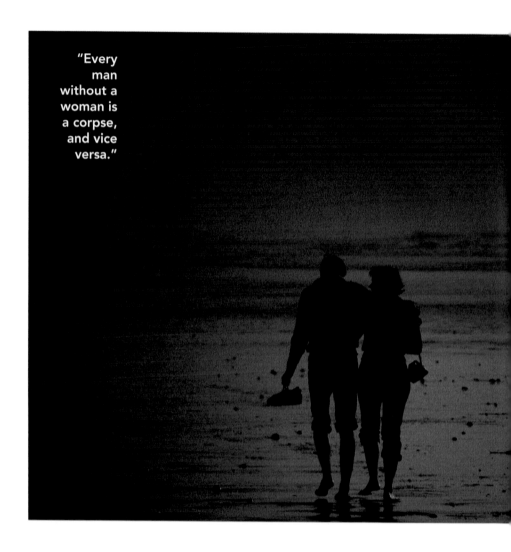

"Every man without a woman is a corpse, and vice versa."

## Tantric couple

A tantric partner is an altar of movement. I learned to live, love, and assess the importance of life and relationships thanks to my Shakti. Any Shiva without his Shakti is a *shava*. Tantra says, "Every man without a woman is a corpse, and vice versa." In the same way that Dali and Gala, Diego Rivera and Frida Kahlo, and so many other couples have a strong fire in their relationship despite storms, I can say that life with a partner means constant learning, maturity, an explosion of experiences, adventures, fires, and warm breezes, and an existential cocktail that makes us constantly learn.

When you have a hardcore partner delivered to you, when you feel you have an ally or a column for holding together the very temple of the relationship, you have a gift from the gods. Walk hand in hand with your partner because it is a miracle, a meditative act. You are with the person you have chosen! Each act of the partner should be loving, docile,

## Use your creative energy through the transformation of sexual energy

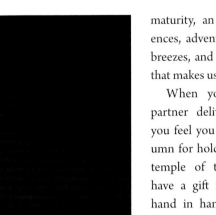

"These three things must be taken into account: the lowest love is sex (physical) and the further refinement of love is compassion. Sex is below love, compassion is above love, and love is exactly in the middle.

Few people know what love is. Unfortunately, a large majority of people believe that sexuality is love, but it is not. Our sexualities are very animalistic, but have the potential to grow into love, but only a potential.

If you have become aware and practice the noble art of meditation, then sex can be transformed into love. If your meditative state becomes full and absolute, then love can be transformed into compassion. Sex is the seed, love is the flower, compassion is the fragrance. Buddha defined compassion as "love plus meditation." When your love is not only a desire for the other, when your love is not the beggar but the emperor, when your love does not ask for anything in return, but is willing to give out of the pure joy of giving . . . throw in the gift of meditation and fragrance will be released. This is compassion. Compassion is the greatest phenomenon."

Osho

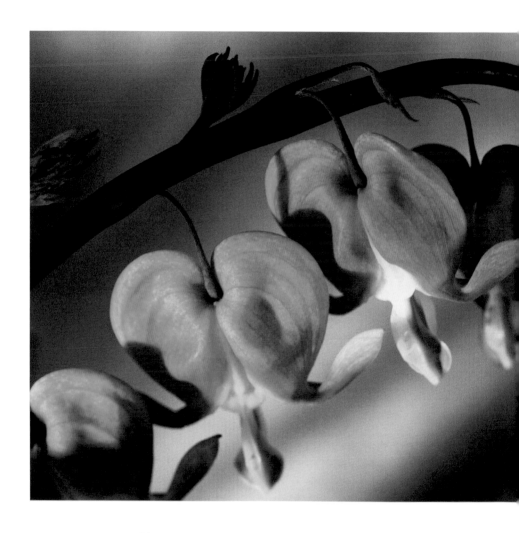

sparkling, nutritious, and provide growth. There are moments of crisis, which are also productive because they give real lessons. You must light candles in order to regain the right direction, become more conscious, become more loving, and become more complete.

Although men are slower to learn (women are infinitely wiser in the field of emotions), I do not change the life of the couple for anything. I think it's a sacred game and an exquisite road of beautiful learning. Women have more respect for the connection and are

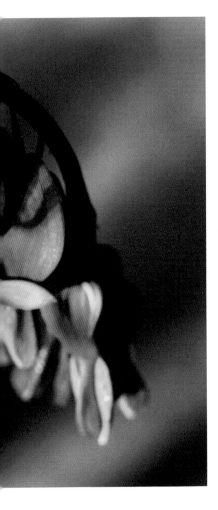

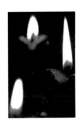

been heavily involved in the use of sexual energy because through it, transformation arises into deep love. Sex is the beginning, the spark of the fire of love. Find the melting point and stay there.

## Don't mortgage your heart

"The heart has reasons that reason does not understand," says a proverb. We are beings who know happiness from the heart and we follow the voice of the heart to be immensely happy, even in moments of suffering. In the balance, when you give your heart and share, you overcome all fear and find the real power of love. The heart is mortgaged when we abandon it, when we create walls, when we give more energy to work than to human beings, when we imagine things that do not exist and are full of fear, when we speculate and censor feelings. We must let love explode. Otherwise, we will feel grey, varying from white to black and never seeing real colors. The heart lives completely in color.

**When you give your heart and share it, you overcome all fear and obtain the true power that is love.**

much deeper than men. For me personally, it took a while to realize this. To wake up each morning next to the love of my life, I feel indivisible, something profoundly magical. Cater to your partner, surprise her, fuel the fire every day because it is the surpreme gift that life gave you. Tantra has

## New tantric "sutras"

The way of Tantra, the path to happiness.

Love, breathe, live.

See each dawn differently.

Generate peace and enthusiasm. Smile. Do not deny or forbid anything.

Be natural; don't speculate. Live without thinking about the clock.

Do not be possessive. Be happy without relying. Appreciate pictures; paint one

Change your hairstyle, be a gardener, dream, search for your destination.

Seduce, trust, shine.

Do not identify yourself, you're just a passenger.

Pray. Keep secrets. Be like a child. Cultivate the spirit.

Take care of your body. Know your desires.

Enjoy. Feel the rain. Sing you what you love. Get creative.

Be attentive and responsive. Let the full moon bewitch you. Change course.

Do not criticize or condemn. Dance erotically. Feel the fire.

Trust yourself. Do not make yourself sick, purify yourself. Imagine positively.

Break routine. Free yourself. Do not control—flow. Use magic.

Live without fear. Do not make barriers: be simple.

Do you know who you are?

Find ecstasy. Do not cling. Do not worry.

Use your touch. Anoint. Be flexible. Let go of sadness.

Do not be divided. Surprise. Live in the present. Raise your energy.

Wake up!

Use awareness, not morality. Do not believe in tradition, look for the cause.

Adapt to the changes. Jump out of the dough. Don't look for security.

Enjoy your work. Roll in the grass. Feel the silence.

Provide service. Fall in love. Pass the tests.

Trust in God.

Do not hurt. Do not repress your feelings. Look at the eyes. Respect your
divinity within.

Relax and do meditation. Defeat laziness. Follow your vocation.

Befriend your loneliness. Look at the sky. Practice yoga.

Connect. Do not let yourself be discredited. Keep your posture.

Express. Do not hold grudges. Be grateful. Love someone.

Open your mind. Do not speak ill of others. Be honest and fun.

Concentrate on giving: we all receive. Sort your stuff.

Close your eyes and look for the mystical.

Enjoy sex with Tantra and the *Kama Sutra*.

Expand yourself. He who makes mistakes, never makes the same twice. Cry. Do not study—learn.

Interpret dreams. Use your power. Don't mark the way. Trust your intuition.

Call on your angel. Take the energy from the sun. Stretch, hit the jump.

Do not accumulate unnecessary things. Have an appointment. Write a poem. Breathe deeply.

Make a gift. Do not carry the past. Be practical.

Sleep eight hours. Work eight hours. Enjoy eight hours.

Say "no" to extremes. Trust the plan. Search for evolution. Do not be mastered.

Do not generate too much expectation. Do not highlight. Cook your food.

Get a massage. Live in secret.

Step into a forest. Do not take everything for granted.

Discover myths. Interpret symbols. Write a letter.

Cultivate telepathy. Love animals.

Light a candle. Think in abundance.

Banish envy. Feel the mystery.

See that the universe has no limits.

Do not worry about things that do not exist. Use your freedom. Do not default on accounts.

Use alchemy. Request discounts. Climb a mountain. Hug a tree.

Be spiritual and material. Do not worry. Do not delay. Keep your pace.

Understand some things well. Do not talk too much. Do not read too much news.

Become wise. Look inside. Do not throw blame.

Take a journey. Play with life.

Become an artist.

Release yourself.

Feel your soul: Enlighten yourself . . . .

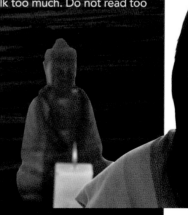

GUILLERMO FERRARA

# Glossary

**Ahamkara.** Individual Ego, the mask of the personality.

**Ajna.** Sixth chakra, third eye, internal capacity to see clearly.

**Amrita.** Feminine ejaculation, liquid with energetic properties.

**Anahatta.** Fourth chakra, relating to emotions and feelings.

**Apana.** Earth energy.

**Asana.** Psychophysical spiritual posture.

**Asvini** Mudra. Anal contraction

**Atma.** Individual soul.

**Atman.** Universal soul.

**Bharata.** Woman invited to share a sexual encounter with a partner.

**Bindu.** Semen.

**Brahma.** God of tantric trilogy, aspect of Creation

**Brahmaranda.** Opening at the top of the head.

**Buddha.** Enlightened state of consciousness.

**Chakra.** Energy wheel that moves the functions of the psyche.

**Chandra.** Moon.

**Chitta.** Unconscious mind.

**Deva.** Sanskrit term for " minor god".

**Dionysus.** Thracian deity who became the Greek representative of ecstasy, trance, and frenzy. Associated with wine and sexual pleasures. The last deity admitted to Olympus. The myth mentions he was born of the muscle (lingam) of Zeus. He was known as Bacchus in Rome, where the sexually initiated women were known as "Bacchae."

**Dwij.** Spiritual rebirth.

**Hatha.** Sun and Moon.

**Harem.** Institution known as "temple of women" or "female sanctuary." Location where a man was with several women.

**Hieros Gamos.** Mystical-sexual ritual known as "sacred marriage" This consists of a group of priestesses and priests practicing the ritual of communion of body and soul reserved for initates into the mysteries of sexuality.

**Ida.** Lunar duct.

**Jalandhara Bhanda.** Jalandhara Bhanda: throat latch to store energy.

**Kali.** Passionate, sensual, and powerful aspect of Shakti, consort of Shiva.

**Kali Yuga.** The Age of Kali (current era).

**Kama Loka.** World of desires.

**Kama Sutra.** Wisdom of desire, Old Hindu treatise concerning the mystical secrets of sexuality.

**Kanda.** Energy oval located under the navel

**Kumbhaka.** Holding one's breath.

**Kundalini.** Sexual and psychic energy stored in the first chakra.

**Laksmi.** Artistic appearance of women, consort of Brahma.

**Lingam.** Male sexual organ.

**Mahamudra.** It means "the great seal or great symbol" and refers to nine seal body orifices together with control of breath and energy.

Performed to understand the nature of the vacuum.

**Maithuna.** Sexual and mystical ritual to feel spiritual transcendence.

**Mandala.** Geometric diagram representing a cross. Tool for meditation.

**Manipura.** Third chakra, solar power

**Mantra.** Spiritual sound to still mind.

**Moksha.** Spiritual liberation.

**Mudra.** Gesture of hands to channel energy.

**Mulabhanda.** Bolt root. Consists of contracting the anal sphincter to stimulate kundalini.

**Muladhara.** First chakra, home of kundalini.

**Nadis.** Conduits along which the vital energy circulates in the energy body.

**Nirvana.** Extinction of ego and fusion of awareness with the ocean of life.

**Ojas Shaktis.** Energy and spiritual power produced by transforming semen.

**Parvati.** Sweet and compassionate aspect of the Shakti.

**Pingala.** Solar duct.

**Pragna.** Intuitive intelligence.

**Prana.** Vital energy.

**Pranayamas.** Techniques to absorb vital energy.

**Puraka.** Inhalation.

**Raja.** Active quality of things.

**Rechacka.** Exhalation.

**Sahasrara.** Seventh chakra, at the top of the head.

**Samadhi.** Consciousness of dissolution, Wholeness.

**Samana.** One of the functions of the prana, linked to excretion.

**Sattva.** Bright and pure quality of things.

**Sexual Magic.** Using sexual energy magically with purpose. The tantric school Vamachara is an old variant of this use. Also well-known magicians such as Aleister Crowley and many esoteric schools as the Gnostics have used this power.

**Shakti.** Energy of the feminine principle.

**Shiva.** God of tantric trinity, energy of the male principle.

**Saraswati.** Consort of Vishnu.

**Siddhis.** Extrasensory powers.

**Surya.** Sun

**Sushumna.** Central tube where kundalini rises.

**Sutras.** Aphorisms, teachings.

**Swadhisthana.** Second chakra, linked with sexual energy.

**Tamas.** Heavy and slow quality of things.

**Udana.** One of the functions of the prana, linked to digestion.

**Uddiyana Bandha.** Upward Abdonminal Lock, for the storage of energy.

**Vayu.** Vital air.

**Vishuda.** Fifth chakra, linked to creativity.

**Vyana.** One of the functions of the prana, which is linked to the circulation of blood.

**Vishnu.** God of tantric trilogy, conservative aspect of nature.

**Yantra.** Visualization technique of figures of power.

**Yoga.** Various energy paths for the conscious integration of the individual with the Cosmos.

**Yoni.** Female sexual organ.

## FINAL NOTE FROM THE AUTHOR

I ask readers to "read" this book with the same spirit with which it was designed. With regard to the nudity, different female models appear because the photographer wanted to reflect in this work and the art of venerating bodies and pleasure in an impersonal form. Many of the photographs were taken on different dates and some match models while others match activities. For the benefit of the work, we wanted to reflect feminine beauty, repressed in the past, as much as possible. The purpose of sexual freedom is to desire more from life. I wanted my priority to be seen as the energy of love (through sex as well as many other ways); this is purely the language of the heart, my heart, which only has room for one magical woman.

## GUILLERMO FERRARA BIOGRAPHY

*Guillermo Ferrara is an artist, therapist, philosopher, and author of twenty-two books and several personal development works. His books have been translated into Spanish, English, Greek, French, Chinese, German, Portuguese, Serbian, Russian, and Romanian. Ferrara is also a researcher of ancient civilizations and ancient cultures. A specialist in holistic philosophy and transpersonal psychology, he teaches about spirituality, Tantra, quantum physics, meditation, yoga, alchemical sexuality, emotional healing, and advances in the field of consciousness, from a spiritual-scientific angle. He has been a Tantra yoga teacher since 1991. Ferrara writes articles for newspapers and is a frequent guest on TV and on the radio. He lives in Miami Beach with his wife, Sandra.*

**Info and Contacts:**
**tantra09@hotmail.com**
**www.guillermoferrara.org**
**www.facebook.com/guillermoferrarainUSA**
**www.twitter.com/GuilleFerrara**